My Child's First Year of Qigong Massage

A Parent Workbook and Companion Volume to

Qigong Massage for Your Child with Autism

by

Louisa Silva

and

Pam Tindall

Qigong Sensory Training Institute

Salem, Oregon

This book is a companion volume to Qigong massage for your child with autism. It is not a substitute and is intended for use in conjunction with it. This book is not a substitute for medical or other professional services. The information contained in this book is intended for educational purposes only.

ISBN 13: 978-0999767900

Library of Congress Control Number: 2015935808

The Qigong Sensory Training Institute (QSTI) is a registered non-profit corporation dedicated to furthering education and research in qigong massage treatment for children with disabilities. Proceeds from the sale of this book will be donated to the Qigong Sensory Training Institute. QSTI Massage and related logos are trademarks belonging to LMT Silva.

First Printing

Front cover design: Paradigm Graphics
Book Design: Sage Waitts

Qigong Sensory Training Institute
Salem, Oregon

Table of Contents

SECTION 1 - GET READY!

What is QST and why is it worth doing?

In this day and age when so many children have problems that cannot be solved with our Western medicine, parents are turning to the wisdom of Eastern medicine for ways to heal their children. And they are finding some beautiful tools. QST massage is such a tool.

What is QST massage for autism? It's a 15-minute, daily, parent-delivered massage for children with autism based on Chinese medicine. And it works for autism.

What does QST stand for? Q is the Chinese medicine part. It stands for qigong – pronounced chee-gong. It is an ancient form of healing that includes massage and movement. It is used to improve health, energy and circulation. **ST** stands for Sensory Treatment. This is a treatment for the sensory problems that stand in the way of development for children with autism.

What does the research show? The research shows that treatment with QST massage results in an average decrease in severity of autism by 32%, sensory problems by 38%, and parenting stress by 44% in the first five months. Continued treatment results in continued benefit. The treatment is an effective sensory treatment for autism. It is started at the time of the autism diagnosis and continued for 1-2 years.

Parents give the massage every day. They learn not to avoid uncomfortable areas, but instead to attune the massage techniques to their children's comfort level. As parents continue the daily massage and work through their children's difficulties, sensory problems diminish. Children start to relax, make eye contact and listen; they become closer and more affectionate with family members. Language and behavior improve. Children ask for their massage, and it is a relaxing, bonding time with their parents.

After five months children's sense of touch is greatly improved, they are better able to regulate behavior,and more comfortable participating in home and school activities. Children with severe autism move towards moderate, moderate children move towards mild, and mild children move off the spectrum. Continued treatment results in continued improvement.

Higher-functioning children make faster progress than lower functioning children because they have more of a foundation for development. Some lower functioning children have cognitive disability and do not learn to speak. It is not possible to identify these children when they are young. Because all children treated with QST massage make sensory, behavioral and social progress, including those who are eventually found to have cognitive disability, we believe all children with autism deserve a chance at this intervention if their parents are willing and able.

Okay, now you know why the massage is worth doing. Let's get set to begin.

Letter to Parents
Introducing the Workbook and
the Year - Long Program

Dear Parents,

QST parent massage is a really different sort of treatment. It's not a medicine. It's not done by a professional. The parent does it. And the parent-child bond makes it more effective. Children respond to their parent's touch like no one else. Parents attune their touch to their children's responses like no one else. And most importantly, parents' love is communicated through touch.

> *"My husband and I do the massage for our son – no outsider can do it better than we can."* Mom

The massage is based on ancient Chinese healing wisdom. This is not a mechanical set of patting and pressing movements. It's true, you have to learn the mechanics of the massage, but that's only the starting point. You also have to learn to read your child's body language during massage and know what to do. You will see where the problems are, attune your touch and work with the problems. Then the massage will help your child get better.

The key to success with this program is you - learning the massage properly and doing it every day for a year. Fifteen minutes a day is what it takes. Ideally, you would have a QST therapist working with you - our research is based on parents having that. But often that is not possible. There are millions of children with autism and not enough QST therapists to go around. If we wait till there are, the children will have grown up.

So we wrote this workbook to give more tools to parents who don't have a therapist - tools to help them understand their child's healing process and keep the massage going day after day for a full year.

The workbook should be used along with the book *Qigong Massage for Your Child With Autism: A Home Program from Chinese Medicine* and DVD. It is not a substitute. The book and DVD are the core of the program. The workbook will help

9

you keep the program going in your family. For instance, you will need to read the book and watch the DVD to learn the 12 movements of the massage before you start, but you'll use the workbook every day to record your observations.

We've learned a lot in the five years since the book was written. We now know more about how parents can maximize their child's success, how to adjust the massage to higher and lower-functioning children, and why the massage works. We'll be sharing what we've learned in the workbook.

If you are like a lot of parents we have worked with, you don't have a lot of extra time. The beauty of this treatment is that it doesn't take a lot of time. It's simple and it works. And you don't have to learn it all at the beginning. You learn some of it at the beginning so that it is possible for you to start. Then you just have to do the massage every day. You learn the rest as you go along. The workbook includes weekly letters from us that will help you build on your learning.

After you get started, you'll see that the massage starts a healing process in your child's body. You might be surprised at how quickly you see small changes. Try to be aware of them. Write them down on the Weekly Logs in the workbook so you'll have a record of your progress. Healing change is good. As you work through the workbook, we'll aim to prepare you in advance for changes that you might see as a result of the massage, and we'll give you massage tools and parenting tips to help.

We've found, after working with hundreds of parents, that after they do the massage for a while, they have questions about things they are seeing in their child and want to learn more. If parents don't get the chance to learn more, they can let the program drop. That's sad because then the child doesn't get the benefit of treatment. That's where we hope the workbook will help. We've included answers to many common questions parents have and some massage solutions.

In **Section 1** of this workbook, you'll see what you need to do before starting your child's program - like reading from the book, and getting yourself and your child ready. We'll also give you a list of goals for yourself - to help you be successful.

In **Section 2** you'll set some goals for the massage, learn why we focus on touch, and discover two tools for measuring your child's progress.

Section 3 is the heart of the workbook. It contains a year's worth of Weekly Logs, alternating with weekly letters to you from us. The Weekly Logs really help you stay on top of the program for the whole year. The letters are your continued learning about the massage. They will tell you what you need to know now, what you can learn later and where you can find additional information. We've also included letters from parents who have done QST massage with their children.

We've written our books so that you don't have to understand Chinese medicine to use the massage effectively. As time passes, you will see what the massage does. If you follow the instructions, it will work. We'll try our best to keep it simple. If you want to know more about the how and why of it, read ahead in the weekly letters.

Section 4 is the Appendices. This section suggests ways to talk with your health care providers and teachers about QST massage.

Section 5 is the index. This section is organized alphabetically so you can look up anything you might have a question about and find useful information. For example, if your child doesn't want you to touch his head during the massage, or she isn't sleeping, you can look up these topics in the index and learn about what this means and what you can do about it.

So here goes, best of luck and enjoy the adventure!

Louisa and Pam

Getting Yourself and Your Support System Ready

Recommended reading: *Qigong Massage for Your Child with Autism: A Home Program from Chinese Medicine* – Chapter 3, "Getting Ready To Give the Home Program"

If possible, two family members should learn the massage. It helps to have two people to share the work and the progress over the year. If one of you is sick or tired, the other one can give the massage on that day and your child won't miss it. If it isn't possible to have another family member help you with the massage, don't worry. Determination makes up for most things. We have seen plenty of single parents do the program solo and have success.

If both parents are living in the same home, and are comfortable with the massage, it is good if they can give the massage together some of the time. According to Chinese medicine, the mother brings the child more nurturing energy (Yin) and the father brings the child more physical strength (Yang) – together it makes for a strong treatment.

Decide where you are going to do the massage, and put the 12-Movement Sheet up on the wall where you can see it while you do massage. It will take you a while to learn the massage by heart.

Goals for Parents

The **starting goal** for you is to learn to give your child a daily massage that is:
1. Done correctly
2. Tuned to your child's body language during massage
3. Tuned to your child's real-life difficulties outside of massage

The more that you can do this, the more effective the massage will be.

The **mid-term goals** are for you to:
1. Learn that your child's responses to touch go through a healing process that goes from under-sensitive to over-sensitive to normal. Recognize where your

child is now, know the signs of shifting to the next stage, and be able to modify the massage accordingly (More about this in Section 2.)

2. Recognize new developmental stages, e.g. the 'terrible twos', and be ready to modify your parenting accordingly

The **final goals** are:

1. For touch to become an easy part of calming and connecting with your child
2. For you to naturally use touch more in your parenting
3. For your child to be closer and more affectionate with you
4. For you both to be able to relax and enjoy the massage together

Are there some parents who cannot achieve these goals?

Almost all parents can learn the massage movements and attune them to their child. Parents naturally stroke, pat and rub their children from the time they are born, and have tons of practice attuning their touch to the child. Parents from all over the world have successfully learned the massage.

Over the years, we have found only a few parents who could not successfully learn to give an attuned massage. These were either:

1. Parents who were on the autism spectrum and had limited sensitivity to touch
2. Parents with neurological problems e.g. seizures, who were on a lot of medication and had limited sensitivity to touch
3. Parents with significant intellectual disability limiting their understanding of the massage process

In these situations, we relied upon the other parent or another adult to give the massage.

Getting your child ready - qigong massage picture storybooks

We have two picture storybooks on our website at www.qsti.org. One is for children with more language and one for children with less. Take a look at both, and use the one that fits best for you and your child. Go through it together several times before starting so you both know what to expect.

SECTION 2 - GET SET!

"It's a lot easier than I thought it was going to be. At first I was like, 'Oh my gosh! I'm not going to be able to learn this massage.' But it's not hard. It really isn't!" Alice M, mother of a five-year-old

Before you begin: Setting goals for the massage

Pick three things you most want the massage to change. Some examples that parents commonly pick are: less tantrums, less aggression, more speech and eating more foods. Pick the three things that are most important to you.

Write in your three goals. It's fun to come back to them after six months, and see what has been accomplished.

1.

2.

3.

Why do we focus on touch?

We focus on touch because touch problems make autism more severe. And if we can treat the touch problems with QST massage, autism gets better and, in some cases, can even go away completely.

When we talk about the sense of touch in children with autism, we are talking about the whole skin and how sensitive it is to being touched - by clothing, a washcloth, or a toothbrush. We pay attention to the skin by area: the back might be fine, but the skin on the hands, head and in the mouth can be over-sensitive, so it can be difficult to trim nails, cut hair, and eat certain foods. We also pay attention to whether the skin is sensitive to injury: does your child show distress when they get hurt? Or do they have a very high pain tolerance? There is a connection between feeling pain and feeling empathy. If a child can't

15

feel pain in their own body, they can't feel empathy for another person's pain.

When we talk about parent touch, we mean the whole-body touch involved in holding, soothing, feeding, and snuggling our child. It is attuned touch - we are very aware of how delicate the baby is. We quickly learn how to support her neck, and how to pat her back to help her get the gas up. This attuned touch is so much a part of caring for children that we don't think about it, we just do it. It brings some of the deepest, most satisfying feelings of closeness, happiness and belonging that we have. Touch is how our children first realize we are here and make eye contact. Who can remember the silent wonder of holding a newborn baby and looking into their eyes? Parent-child touch is the first touch that brings those feelings of deep, calm connection. It feels so good, we long for it and keep coming back for more. That's why children seek connection.

In autism, research shows that children have problems with touch - it doesn't feel so good. Children might withdraw from touch, or they might not notice it. Some areas of the body might feel okay, but other areas hurt with even light touch, and yet other areas are numb when injured. It's a very confusing picture of the body for the child's brain, and this patchwork of different feelings makes it hard for the child to develop a whole sense of self. As a result, there is no way that parent touch can work in the same way as it does in typically developing children. In autism, touch doesn't calm children down, and children don't seek it out as much for comfort and reassurance.

What happens with the massage is that it steadily reverses the problem with touch. First, massage brings children an awareness of their bodies and themselves. Then massage begins to bring normal feeling back to the skin. Over the first six months, the numb areas wake up, and the over-sensitive areas calm down. Children start to get a sense of self, and you see the independent little person come out. As feeling returns, children naturally show empathy. And the best part is that children seek out touch again because parent touch calms and reassures them. By the end, children can come out of their separate world and join our world more.

"The shell that was around him has dropped off, And he has light!"
Mother, 4 year old

Let's take a look at graphs showing the before-and-after progress from five months of daily parent massage and you will see the one-to-one connection between touch and behavior.

Progress with 5 Months of QST Massage

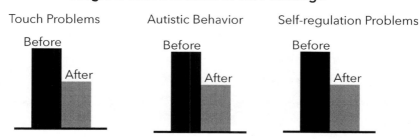

Notice that when touch problems go down, autistic behavior goes down too. That is because the problems with touch drive the problems with behavior. It's cause and effect. The massage treats the cause.

Also notice the last two bars - self-regulation problems. Parents' eyes often glaze over when we mention wanting to improve self-regulation. That is until they realize what it is. Then it is "Oh, do I want my child to sleep through the night? Yes, definitely!" "Do I want the diarrhea and constipation to stop? Yes, absolutely!" "Do I want the tantrums to stop? Yes!" "Do I want her to make eye contact and pay attention when I talk to her? Yes, I would love that!" The self-regulation milestones are about being able to regulate the really important things:

Sleep - sleeping through the night

Digestion - eating a variety of foods and digesting well

Behavior - being able to handle change and transitions without getting upset

Attention - being able to pay attention to, look at, listen to and learn from other people

"I've only been doing the massage for a week and already he's sleeping better. That means I am, too!" - Mom

"She's started feeding herself and doesn't spit out new foods like she used to." - Father

"He's able to calm himself down much easier. He hardly has any major tantrums any more." - Mother

"Every hour I've put into this massage with my son has been paid back to me in full when he looks at me and smiles!" - Mother

So, you can see why self-regulation milestones are important. They make development of healthy bodies and minds possible, and they are delayed in children with autism. Parent touch helps to put self-regulation milestones in place in typically developing children, and the massage helps put them in place in children with autism.

Looking at the graphs, you'll notice that the self-regulation problems improve almost as much as the touch problems do. There is a one-to-one connection there, too. We pay attention to sleep, digestion, attention and behavior in the Weekly Logs - these things improve too, and they will help your child grow and develop normally.

Do I have to do the massage every day?

QST massage must be given every day in the first half of the year in order to be effective. Your child's sensory system has been out of kilter for some years, and his brain and body have been in an autistic pattern of growth and development. You can change that with the massage, but only if you do it every day. The research shows it just doesn't work as well if you let the frequency fall to every other day. When the body and brain have been stuck in a pattern, it takes time, effort and energy to change that pattern. That is what you are doing with the massage. You are forming a new pattern. You are giving your child the chance to improve the way he or she takes in sensory information and learns.

Each time you work through a difficult area on your child's body, and come out on the other side to where he can now tolerate touch on that area without difficulty, you have given a huge gift to your child. In the end, you will have given him the ability to feel comfortable just being himself. With that gift he can enjoy cuddling with you, he can recover his curiosity, and he can enjoy playing with other children. No one can give that gift like a parent can.

You will also be teaching your child's nervous system to relax. That, too, takes time. The nervous system of a child with autism is easily stressed and overwhelmed. The usual ways of reassuring and calming the child – parent touch – don't work very well. As you bring your child's sense of touch back to normal, his nervous system will relax more and more. At the end of the day, no matter what the difficulties of the day, you will be able to give a massage that will bring your child's nervous system back into balance so that he can learn and grow from his experiences. After six months of daily massage, the research shows that the new pattern will have emerged. After that, you want to keep doing the massage 5-7 times a week to maintain progress.

> *"Qigong massage gives us tools to calm our child and has become a part of our bedtime routine. It helps him calm down and be able to sleep. " - Mom*

> *"Our family was on vacation for a weekand our son would not let a day go by without us doing the massage before bed. It's just what we do now." - Dad*

> *"It's brought us all closer. It's good for our kids and it's good for us, too!" - Parents*

How you will measure progress

There are lots of ways to measure progress. One way is to have a gut sense of it - some parents are fine with that. Another way is to set goals like you just did, go back to them in six months, see how many have been reached, and set new goals. Some parents prefer this. A third way is to use two simple tests - the Autism Touch/Pain Checklist, and the Autism Parenting Stress Index. The first test evaluates how severe the touch/pain abnormality is, and the second evaluates how difficult it is to parent your child. If you use these tests, you can watch how the scores change over the year. This is a great way to track progress, since sometimes we're just so busy parenting that we can miss little improvements and how they add up to big improvements over time. If you are up for it, we recommend that you do all three.

When QST trainers work with parents, they have parents fill out the two tests at the beginning, middle and end of the year. They are looking for the scores to come down to where typical children score. Depending on how severe the child's autism is to begin with, this can take a year or two. Children with more severe autism change more slowly at first, and can take months to recover the basics like making eye contact and being able to calm down, focus and listen. Children with milder autism make faster progress. They already have somewhat of a foundation to build on, but their social foundation needs work - they need to learn to enjoy physical and emotional closeness with other people.

Therapists use the scores to measure progress and advise parents how long to continue the intervention. If the scores improve by 10% in the first half of the year, we can be pretty sure that at the end of the year they will improve by 20% if the parent does the daily massage. It may not be as fast as the parent wants, but it is still a sizable gain, and will make a big difference for the child. If scores are improved by 25% at mid-year, we can be fairly certain that at the end of the year they will improve by 50% if the parent does the daily massage. We can't control the speed of healing, but once we see it is happening, we can celebrate it!

So, for this year, we will give you the opportunity to go the goal-setting route and to go the testing route. The testing is definitely quick and easy. It takes less than 15 minutes. But please be accurate when you fill out the answers - you will want an accurate measure of progress due to all your work!

Autism Touch/Pain Checklist

Circle the response for each item that most accurately describes your child.

1. **Touch/Pain**	Often	Sometimes	Rarely	Never
• Does not cry tears when hurt	3	2	1	0
• Doesn't notice if the diaper is wet or dirty	3	2	1	0
• Face washing is difficult	3	2	1	0
• Haircuts are difficult	3	2	1	0
• Refuses to wear a hat	3	2	1	0
• Prefers to wear a hat	3	2	1	0
• Cutting fingernails is difficult	3	2	1	0
• Prefers to wear one or two gloves	3	2	1	0
• Avoids wearing gloves	3	2	1	0
• Cutting toenails is difficult	3	2	1	0
• Will only wear certain footwear (e.g. soft shoes, no socks)	3	2	1	0
• Prefers to wear the same clothes day after day	3	2	1	0
• Will only wear certain clothes (e.g. no elastic, no tags, only short pants)	3	2	1	0
• Cries tears when falls, scrapes skin or gets hurt (scale is reversed on purpose)	0	1	2	3
• Head bangs on a hard surface	3	2	1	0
• Head bangs on a soft surface	3	2	1	0
Add up the scores in each column:	___	___	___	___

Add up the total score: _____

The Autism Parenting Stress Index

Please rate the following aspects of your child's health **according to how much stress it causes you and/or your family** by placing an X in the box that best describes your situation.	Not stressful	Sometimes creates stress	Often creates stress	Very stressful on a daily basis	So stressful at times I feel I cannot cope
Your child's ability to communicate					
Tantrums/meltdowns					
Aggressive behavior (siblings, peers)					
Self-injurious behavior					
Difficulty making transitions from one activity to another					
Sleep problems					
Your child's diet					
Bowel problems (diarrhea, constipation)					
Potty training					
Not feeling close to your child					
Concern for the future of your child being accepted by others					
Concern for the future of your child living independently					

Subtotal: _____ _____ _____ _____ _____

Total: _____

Letter to Parents – Anna's Story

Dear parents,

When we started this, my daughter was three, and she didn't have any language. She was kind of in her own world. It was really hard to start the massage. She would get overwhelmed, and we would have to do bits of the massage at a time, and use my phone to distract her. Gradually over the first few months, she got used to it, and got to where I could give her the whole massage without using my phone.

Now we have given it to her every day for two years. It's a relaxing, bonding time for us. I've always been 'her person', but we are even closer now. She has become really social. She loves her big sister. She goes into her room when she wants her to play with her. And her big sister loves playing with her. Her language has come a long way too. She understands everything, and she talks when she wants to.

My daughter is doing really well in preschool. The teachers tell me they are really happy with how she is doing. They told me she met all her goals, and now they have increased her goals. I observed in her classroom, and it brought me to tears when I saw how much she was engaging with the teachers and wanting to do things. It used to be that we would sit in the parking lot and she would cry, and I would comfort her. Now she isn't even upset when she goes to school. Now she goes right in, and is happy to be there.

Before we started the massage, her testing put her in the severe autism range, and now when they just tested her, she doesn't even make the "mild autism" cutoff! Yes, she still has developmental delays, but she is learning and growing every day. We are thinking that she can be in mainstream kindergarten next year. The massage has been a very important part of her progress, and I recommend it.

Sincerely,

Anna's Mom

SECTION 3: GO!

Weekly Logs - stay the course

For each week of your year of Qigong massage, you will find in this workbook a personal letter to you and a Weekly Log.

The personal letters to you will be from the two of us – Louisa and Pam – or possibly from another parent, family member or qigong therapist. In these letters we will share information we think you can use that week.

Early in the year we'll talk about learning the massage, dealing with any resistance you might find, what to look for, and how to adjust the massage to your child's responses. A bit later we'll offer some extra techniques and talk a little more deeply about how Qigong massage works to address some common problems for children with autism. Later we'll talk about shifting your parenting techniques to match your child's new development and how you can talk with your child's teacher and doctor about QST. Finally, you'll hear from other parents and therapists about their experiences.

These letters are designed to anticipate what we think you will need as you move through the year of qigong massage. We think they will help keep you motivated to "stay the course" when life gets hectic, the routine gets a little dull or you need a weekly pep talk. We think you'll find the letters from other parents especially enjoyable.

The Weekly Log is where you mark down every day you give the massage and write notes. We strongly encourage you write your thoughts, feelings, observations and changes every single week on your Weekly Logs. This will help you keep track of progress, changes, challenges, improvements others are noticing, and questions you have that you may want to look up in the book. It will be a very helpful tool for your child's IEP, therapists, doctor or teacher, as well, as you all work together. We printed one Weekly Log for every week because we think it's that important. We hope you'll use it every week.

Week 1

Letter to parents - Learning the massage: Patting and pressure

Recommended Reading: *Qigong Massage for Your Child With Autism: A Home Program from Chinese Medicine,* Chapter 4 and watch the DVD.

Dear parents,

OK. You've done the recommended reading and watched the DVD. You've practiced the massage and you are reasonably comfortable with the 12 movements. You've pinned the 12 movement sheet to the wall where you are going to give the massage so you can see it. And you've filled out the Autism Touch/Pain and Parenting Stress Checklists.

Now comes the most important part of this massage and what makes it different. It has to be attuned to your child's responses. This is not a one-size-fits-all treatment. And your emotions are really important. You have to be calm. Your child will feel your calmness and it will help him during the massage.

When starting movements 1 and 2, you'll have to figure out what kind of touch - patting or pressing - to start with. How will you know? It's not so hard - you are already tuned in to your child, and it's easy for you to tell what they like and don't like.

Answering the following question will help you figure it out: Does your child have a high pain tolerance when he is hurt?

If your answer is yes - your child may be more on the under-sensitive side and you will probably need to start with patting. Patting opens up awareness of the skin.

If your answer is no - your child might be on the over-sensitive side - aware of touch but unable to handle much of it. You will probably have to start with pressing. Pressing improves tolerance to touch.

Either way, regardless of what "most children" like - you'll need to pick the technique that works best for your child.

The basic idea is this. In general, children who are under-sensitive have less awareness and tend to have less language. They usually need a lot of patting on the head and back of the body to open up awareness. One sign that they are opening up is if they start humming while you are patting. After a few months they often make a switch to being over-sensitive. Be on the look-out for it because then they will want you to switch to pressing, and it will help them feel the different parts of their body come together as a whole.

In general, children who are over-sensitive have more awareness and more language. They are aware of touch but unable to handle much of it. You will probably have to start with pressing. Pressing improves tolerance to touch. When they can tolerate patting, you'll know their skin is returning to normal.

Don't worry if you don't understand it all at first. It's a lot to grasp. An ancient form of natural healing for a modern childhood disability! You will be working on it for a whole year, and by the end of that time, you'll understand a lot!

Our very best wishes for your journey,

Louisa and Pam

Weekly Log - Week 1

♥ Always start with love

Check each day you do the massage

Sun ___ Mon ___ Tuesday ___ Wed ___ Thu ___ Fri ___ Sat ___

Things You Noticed:

During the Massage

Mv1. Lays down/won't lay down?

Mv2. Back – hums?

Mv3-4. Ears – avoids?

Mv5. Up/up/up – eye contact?

Mv6. Fingers – stroking or pressing?

Mv7. Chest – rubs eyes, yawns, relaxes?

Mv8. Belly – diarrhea/constipation?

Mv9-10. Legs – patting or pressing?

Mv11. Toes – stroking, pressing, bicycle?

Mv12. Soles – avoids?

During the Week

Sleep _____

Bowels _____

Tantrums _____

Affection _____

Eye contact _____

Listening _____

Speaking _____

Other_____

Positive things other people said about your child ...

Your thoughts and feelings about the process ...

Questions you had this week ...

Remember: Look for answers to your questions in the index and the book.

Week 2

Letter to Parents - Working with Resistance to massage

Dear Parents,

When first starting massage, there are quite a few children who resist or refuse it. If this is your child, you can feel reassured in the fact that most children accept it pretty quickly. What you don't want to do is force the massage on your child, or get into a struggle with him over massage - this will not work. After all, the basic principle behind the massage is to help your child relax and connect! We want him to have his daily treatment, and we have to find a way for him to tolerate it until massage improves his response to touch.

> *"When we started the massage, we found it pretty difficult for a few weeks. Our son would complain that his body hurt. But pretty soon he started to enjoy the massage. Then the changes started – he slept and ate better, played on his own and his language got a lot clearer. It was so worth sticking with it through those first hard weeks." - Mother*

Many parents have discovered that one of the best things to do if their child is resisting is to use TV or video to occupy his attention while they give the massage. First, figure out whether you want to start with patting or pressing. Then get him involved in a video, calmly sit next to him, and start the massage. In this situation, you will not be able to go for eye contact in Movement 5 - that will be later. For now, you will be aiming to get through the massage and start his skin feeling better so he'll resist less.

After several weeks, or even a few months in some cases, you can try to wean him away from video during the massage. Start with him watching a video on your phone, and then if his eyes leave the video, slowly turn it over. When he wants it back, turn it back. You will notice that over time, his attention will wander away from the video more and more. We have found that eventually even the children who resist the massage the most at the beginning don't need video to get through the massage. Once you are not using video, you can go for eye contact in

Movement 5.

You might think your child should start the massage by lying down, but he might not be ready to do that. You might have to start the massage with him standing or sitting. This is not a problem - we start where the child is. Don't worry, the massage will first help you to take care of the problem with touch, later you will get the relaxation. If he is moving around, it will help to contain him in front of the TV in the arms of the other parent. You should not restrain him; this will cause him to struggle. But there is a way to contain him within your widespread arms, and keep him within reach while the other parent does the massage.

While some children might resist the massage completely at first, some parents have found that their child tolerates the first few minutes of massage fine, but then gets overwhelmed and wants to stop. If you notice your child is getting overwhelmed, take a short break (about one minute) and then go back and pick up the massage where you left off. Don't let the break be so long that your child gets off the table and gets involved in another activity. But short breaks help some children tolerate the massage for longer and longer, and the 'overwhelm' usually disappears within a few weeks.

> *"She still resists some, but is getting a little calmer during the massage. She can tolerate movements 1 and 2 now, and sometimes movements 3 and 4 before we have to take a little break. So that's progress!"- Father*

Keep up the good work. Resistance is just a phase that your child will pass through. If you stick with it, the massage really will improve his enjoyment of touch, and your enjoyment of this very special time together.

Best wishes,

Louisa and Pam

Weekly Log - Week 2

♥ Always start with love

Check each day you do the massage

Sun ___ Mon ___ Tuesday ___ Wed ___ Thu ___ Fri ___ Sat ___

Things You Noticed:

During the Massage

Mv1. Lays down/won't lay down?

Mv2. Back – hums?

Mv3-4. Ears – avoids?

Mv5. Up/up/up – eye contact?

Mv6. Fingers – stroking or pressing?

Mv7. Chest – rubs eyes, yawns, relaxes?

Mv8. Belly – diarrhea/constipation?

Mv9-10. Legs – patting or pressing?

Mv11. Toes – stroking, pressing, bicycle?

Mv12. Soles – avoids?

During the Week

Sleep _____

Bowels _____

Tantrums _____

Affection _____

Eye contact _____

Listening _____

Speaking _____

Other_____

Positive things other people said about your child ...

Your thoughts and feelings about the process ...

Questions you had this week ...

Remember: Look for answers to your questions in the index and the book.

Week 3

Letter to Parents – Signs you will see during massage

Recommended Reading: *Qigong Massage for Your Child With Autism: A Home Program from Chinese Medicine*, Chapter 5

Dear Parents,

In a way, what you are doing with the massage is making up for what your child wouldn't let you do when she was smaller. She wouldn't let you hold her to calm her down and put her to sleep. And if you did hold her in your arms, she wouldn't look you in the eyes and pay attention to you.

Now she's older and she still hasn't learned to put herself to sleep, calm herself down, or look you in the eyes. She hasn't learned those things because a child's brain needs lots and lots of positive, reassuring, calming parent touch to learn those things, and touch hasn't been positive, reassuring and calming for her. If she is like a lot of children with autism, she doesn't like touch a whole lot, and she has some areas of real discomfort and numbness on her skin.

The beauty of the QST massage is that you are going to find the skin areas that are uncomfortable and make them feel better: numb areas are going to wake up, uncomfortable areas are going to calm down, and both are going to be able to feel good.

> *"I loved that the massage helped him be comfortable in his own body. It allowed my son to experience touch in a positive manner, which allowed him to experience other emotions, too. This has been a spectacular experience." - Mom*

Over the first six months, you will find every area that is uncomfortable and work with it until it is comfortable. The astonishing thing is that the very areas that are uncomfortable need to be comfortable in order for development to proceed normally. For example, if the skin on his ears is uncomfortable, a child will avoid everything about his ears, including listening. Once you use QST massage to make the ears feel normal, he will stop avoiding his ears and start using them to listen.

A similar thing happens with fingers. One of the first steps for early communication is pointing - the child points to what she wants. They call it gestural language. But if the fingers are uncomfortable, she will avoid touch on her fingers, and she won't use them to point. Gestural language never gets out of the starting gate. But you are going to massage her fingers until they are comfortable. This will take a month or less. Once they are comfortable, she will start using them to point. And then you will see something amazing during her massage: you will see evidence of the direct connection between the fingers (early gestural language) and the speech area of the brain. After a few minutes of massaging her fingers, you will see her lips and tongue start moving. She will not be aware of it, and you do not need to draw her attention to it, but you will have activated the speech area of her brain. You will have jumpstarted speech. You will continue to massage the fingers a few minutes longer, and can expect some new language in the days and weeks to come.

When something isn't working in your house, you determine where it is broken, fix it, and then check to see if it is working again. In the process, you follow two kinds of signs - signs that it isn't working, and signs that it is working. QST massage is a similar process. As you go through the 12 movements, your child will show you by his reactions where the problems are. Where things hurt is important. It tells you the areas of skin that aren't working (sensing normally) and need to be fixed. Then you use the massage to 'fix' those areas.

Three signs the skin isn't sensing normally

Pain:

When a certain area is uncomfortable, your child will pull away from your hand, or try to pull your hand away. Remember, it's not normal for the massage to hurt! It means you have just found a place that needs treatment. The most common areas where children are uncomfortable are ears, fingers and toes, but other areas show up too.

What do you do to fix it? You stay on the area and switch to the opposite technique. If you are patting, you switch to pressing; if you are pressing you switch to patting. You continue for a while and observe whether your child relaxes. The sign that she is uncomfortable should stop, then you can continue on with the massage. Fingers can take a month to get better. Ears can take longer, especially if there is a severe speech delay, and toes take the longest, sometimes several months.

Ticklishness:

A common sign of ticklishness is giggling. The neck, fingers, toes or legs can be ticklish. When the neck is ticklish, you will see your child hunching their shoulders and giggling when you massage it. Ticklishness is a sign that the skin is over-sensitive. When you see the sign, stay on the area, but slow down and switch to pressing. Continue for a while, the sign should stop. Remember to look for it next time – it is often gone in a few days.

Numbness:

You don't see this sign during massage. You see it when your child falls and hurts himself, and doesn't cry. What you see in massage is what happens when numbness suddenly goes away and is replaced with something else - your child who has been calmly letting you do the massage for weeks or months, suddenly acts like it hurts. And he acts different the rest of the time – he seems to be over-stimulated. This is something that happens in at least half the children we have worked with – he has entered the hypersensitivity phase.

"He said he felt a cut on his thumb and asked for a bandaid! This was new." - Father

"He feels his hands when they are cold now and will wear his mittens." - Mother

"She can feel pain now. She's also stopped biting me and actively hugs me. Qigong works!" - Mom

Your child's skin, which has been numb, has started feeling again. He is now way more aware of his body than he was before, and he is adjusting to all the new sensations. You can make a huge difference with massage if you recognize this phase. You should immediately switch all the movements to pressing. Don't move the skin much - just press gently in and out, as you follow down the movements. The pressing will increase his tolerance to touch, and calm down his nervous system. Within a few weeks the phase will pass, touch will feel good, he will feel normal pain in response to injury, he will feel empathy, and he will be more cuddly and affectionate. What wonderful rewards for making it through the hypersensitivity phase!

Keep up the good work!

Louisa and Pam

Weekly Log - Week 3

♥ Always start with love

Check each day you do the massage

Sun ___ Mon ___ Tuesday ___ Wed ___ Thu ___ Fri ___ Sat ___

Things You Noticed:

During the Massage

Mv1. Lays down/won't lay down?

Mv2. Back – hums?

Mv3-4. Ears – avoids?

Mv5. Up/up/up – eye contact?

Mv6. Fingers – stroking or pressing?

Mv7. Chest – rubs eyes, yawns, relaxes?

Mv8. Belly – diarrhea/constipation?

Mv9-10. Legs – patting or pressing?

Mv11. Toes – stroking, pressing, bicycle?

Mv12. Soles – avoids?

During the Week

Sleep _____

Bowels _____

Tantrums _____

Affection _____

Eye contact _____

Listening _____

Speaking _____

Other_____

Positive things other people said about your child ...

Your thoughts and feelings about the process ...

Questions you had this week ...

Remember: Look for answers to your questions in the index and the book.

Week 4
Letter to Parents - Signs the massage is working

Recommended Reading: *Qigong Massage for Your Child With Autism: A Home Program from Chinese Medicine*, Chapter 6

Dear Parents,

When we said the skin was connected to the brain by millions of tiny sensory nerves, we really meant it. Somehow we tend to think of the brain as something that is locked away inside the skull. We forget about the millions of sensory nerves that connect it to every square inch of skin. Why are all those connections there? Because touch makes the brain grow. And touch is how we learn to be social.

Human beings are social animals - we survive by being social. But we are not born knowing how to be social. We have to learn how. We learn how to eat, sleep, care for ourselves, communicate, get along, and live together from other people. And in the early years, the child is rewarded for being social every step of the way.

Pleasure and satisfaction are the reward. In those first years when touch is the dominant sense, touch brings pleasure and satisfaction every time a child is fed and cared for. And each time he is fed and cared for, he faces his parent and sees his pleasure and satisfaction mirrored in his parent's face. Touch makes the physical connection that gives the feeling of closeness and triggers the eye contact that allows feelings to be shared.

When we make eye contact with our child, we have the feeling that we are in contact with the mind of our child and we can know his mind. It's quite amazing when you think about it!

A lot of this has been missing for children with autism because of the difficulties with touch and eye contact. Parents have longed for it, but have not been able to make it happen. Now you can. It is your job, not only to help your child's skin to feel good again, but to start up those skin/brain connections that have been dormant.

Here's how you know the skin-brain connections are starting up. There are signs. Some of these signs look really normal. And they are, until you realize that they are things your child does not normally do in response to touch. And some of them are things you've never seen before. Here is the short list:

He relaxes with touch. These signs happen in progressive stages when you massage the head and back during Movements 1 and 2:

- He stops struggling with touch/massage
- He lies down when massage starts
- He puts his head down
- He relaxes his body

He connects with his own body and with you

- Humming - he is connecting with his body and enjoying massage. This sign usually happens with the back, Movements 1 and 2
- Making eye contact - he is connecting with you. This sign usually happens with the arm and hand, Movements 5 and 6
- Smiling at you - he is communicating his pleasure. This sign usually happens with the arm and hand, Movements 5 and 6

He self-soothes. Now his brain is self-regulating towards deep relaxation. This sign usually happens with the chest (Movement 7)

- Closing the eyes
- Rubbing the eyes
- Yawning

Parts of his brain that have been asleep are activated. This sign usually happens with fingers (Movement 6):

- Spontaneous movements of the lips and tongue - the speech area of the brain is activating

His brain integrates the new information. This sign usually happens with movement 12.

- Small twitching movements of the eyes and face - the brain is making connections and integrating

These signs all mean that the information contained in the massage is reaching your child's brain and teaching him basic social and self-regulation skills: how to relax, connect, communicate, stay calm and feel good together. You can be very happy when you see these signs. Because once massage helps his brain make the connection, it will help him regulate his behavior and be more social in daily life.

This is good work you're doing,

All our best,

Louisa and Pam

Weekly Log - Week 4

♥ Always start with love

Check each day you do the massage

Sun ___ Mon ___ Tuesday ___ Wed ___ Thu ___ Fri ___ Sat ___

Things You Noticed:

During the Massage

Mv1. Lays down/won't lay down?

Mv2. Back – hums?

Mv3-4. Ears – avoids?

Mv5. Up/up/up – eye contact?

Mv6. Fingers – stroking or pressing?

Mv7. Chest – rubs eyes, yawns, relaxes?

Mv8. Belly – diarrhea/constipation?

Mv9-10. Legs – patting or pressing?

Mv11. Toes – stroking, pressing, bicycle?

Mv12. Soles – avoids?

During the Week

Sleep _____

Bowels _____

Tantrums _____

Affection _____

Eye contact _____

Listening _____

Speaking _____

Other_____

Positive things other people said about your child ...

Your thoughts and feelings about the process ...

Questions you had this week ...

Remember: Look for answers to your questions in the index and the book.

Week 5

Letter to Parents – Getting comfortable with the massage, noticing more

Dear Parents,

Well, you've passed the four-week mark, now. You've given the massage almost 30 times, and hopefully it's closer to becoming second nature to you. One of the things parents say to us at the end of our program is:

> *"The massage seems so natural to me. It's how I touch my child anyway." - Kari M, mother*

If you've ever really looked at a mom playing with her six month child on her lap, you'll see she is constantly touching him, stroking him, playing with his hands and feet, kissing him, rubbing him, facing him in towards her, facing him out towards the people in the room. Try observing it sometime. You'll be amazed! In a single hour, the mom will touch her baby thousands of times. Yet if somebody had walked by and looked, all they would have seen was a mom playing with her baby - nothing unusual at all. It is really natural for us to touch our children - a lot.

Once you and your child are more used to the massage itself, you'll find yourself relaxing into it. Parents tell us that they may start the massage tired from the activities of the day, but after massage, they feel refreshed. Massage helps both of you. That's actually what the massage research shows - that massage relaxes the person giving the massage almost as much as the person receiving it.

When it is the parent giving massage, the effects are even stronger because touch releases bonding hormones in both of you. Almost every parent who has done our program reports that the massage brought their child closer to them.

> *"The massage brought us closer. He is much more affectionate and cuddly, now." - Mary J, mother*

As you relax into the massage process more, your own senses will open up, and you'll notice things. You'll become more aware of your child's body, and you'll find "trouble-spots", especially around his neck and under his ears. Don't be afraid to work on them as you go along - tap them lightly with your fingertips, or press them gently in and out depending which he prefers or tolerates better.

Another thing parents sometimes notice during the first few months of massage is strange smells and tastes.

> "When I did his massage last week, I could taste something in my mouth that seemed metallic". - Andrew C, father

This means that the massage is helping your child's body get rid of toxins he may have taken in from his food or the environment. If the taste or smell gets too strong, just open a window, and keep going. As your child relaxes, his circulation improves, and it is not unusual for his body to start flushing out in the first few months of massage. Research shows that children with autism have higher levels of chemicals in their bodies than other children. It is good for your child to flush that stuff out. Massage helps.

Another thing that parents wonder about is whether there is anything qigong can do for them. Caring for a child with autism can be wearing. And yes, there is. People in China have done qigong exercises to improve health and vitality for thousands of years. These exercises really work if you do them every day. Research shows that they decrease stress, improve energy and strengthen the immune system. We have created a 15-minute qigong exercise routine especially for our parents and therapists. If you are interested in this for yourself, you can take a look at the bookstore on our website. If you have the time to do it every day, we promise you, you won't be sorry.

Keep up the good work – you'll both come out of this at the other end being healthier and more "in touch" with yourselves.

All the best,
Louisa and Pam

Weekly Log - Week 5

♥ Always start with love

Check each day you do the massage

Sun ___ Mon ___ Tuesday ___ Wed ___ Thu ___ Fri ___ Sat ___

Things You Noticed:

During the Massage

Mv1. Lays down/won't lay down?

Mv2. Back – hums?

Mv3-4. Ears – avoids?

Mv5. Up/up/up – eye contact?

Mv6. Fingers – stroking or pressing?

Mv7. Chest – rubs eyes, yawns, relaxes?

Mv8. Belly – diarrhea/constipation?

Mv9-10. Legs – patting or pressing?

Mv11. Toes – stroking, pressing, bicycle?

Mv12. Soles – avoids?

During the Week

Sleep _____

Bowels _____

Tantrums _____

Affection _____

Eye contact _____

Listening _____

Speaking _____

Other_____

Positive things other people said about your child ...

Your thoughts and feelings about the process ...

Questions you had this week ...

Remember: Look for answers to your questions in the index and the book.

Week 6

Parent Letter – Parent Support Hands and how to include your other children

Dear Parents,

You've been giving qigong massage to your child now for a while, and the two of you have probably settled into a nice routine and are enjoying this special time together. Your child is probably tolerating a lot more touch by now, so it's a great time to share this with the rest of the family – your parenting partner, other adults in the family or your other children. Remember how important touch is to children's development? Children get so many benefits from many-hands massage!

There are so many ways to invite your parenting partner, other family adults or other children to join in. You can alternate repetitions of each movement or work together in each one. For example, in movements 1 and 2, one parent can pat down the head and back and another family member can pick up the movement at the hips and pat down the lower body to the heels. Especially if your child is having a hard time staying down for the massage or her feet are floating up or her legs are kicking, this will help bring your child's energy down.

In movement 3, especially if your child has had a lot of ear infections, having one person pat the ear while another pats on top of the shoulder can really help clear out the ears. A third person can even join in by patting down the sides of the body! In movement 4, a similar approach can be taken with the second person patting or pressing down the arms. With movements 5 and 6, it's often helpful for a second person to gently place their hand on the child's chest for social and language support.

In general when working on the upper body, a support hand on the chest is wonderful; when working on the lower body, a support hand on the belly is good. Even very young children in the family can participate in this way.

If your child has constipation, it can be helpful for a second person to pat down the front of his legs while one parent does the belly circles in movement 8.

In the case of diarrhea, have the second person press down the front of the child's legs instead of patting. Finally, while one parent is doing movements 10 and 11, a support hand on the lower belly will help the child's body make a connection between her belly and her lower legs and help her gross motor skills advance.

Any time during the massage, but especially once you get to movement 12, support hands on your child's chest and belly really help her body stabilize and integrate the entire massage. Sometimes children will take a parent's hand and lay it on their forehead or face, chest or belly. If you're attuned to their responses, they will often show you just how to use your support hands!

Many hands not only make light work, in this case they boost the effectiveness of the massage and bring the family close. Enjoy!

All our best,

Louisa and Pam

Weekly Log - Week 6

♥ Always start with love

Check each day you do the massage

Sun ___ Mon ___ Tuesday ___ Wed ___ Thu ___ Fri ___ Sat ___

Things You Noticed:

During the Massage

Mv1. Lays down/won't lay down?

Mv2. Back – hums?

Mv3-4. Ears – avoids?

Mv5. Up/up/up – eye contact?

Mv6. Fingers – stroking or pressing?

Mv7. Chest – rubs eyes, yawns, relaxes?

Mv8. Belly – diarrhea/constipation?

Mv9-10. Legs – patting or pressing?

Mv11. Toes – stroking, pressing, bicycle?

Mv12. Soles – avoids?

During the Week

Sleep _____

Bowels _____

Tantrums _____

Affection _____

Eye contact _____

Listening _____

Speaking _____

Other_____

Positive things other people said about your child ...

Your thoughts and feelings about the process ...

Questions you had this week ...

Remember: Look for answers to your questions in the index and the book.

Week 7

Letter to parents – An extra technique to make transitions easy

Recommended Reading: *Qigong Massage for Your Child With Autism: A Home Program from Chinese Medicine*, Chapter 7

Dear Parents,

By now your child is used to the massage and calms down much quicker with your touch and your voice. You are able to trigger self-soothing in him when you do Movement 7 and his tantrums are fewer, shorter and less intense.

But he may still have some difficulties making transitions. For example, it's time to stop playing and get on the table for massage. Even though he likes massage, he resists your instructions. He feels you are taking something away from him. Change isn't easy for him, and he needs extra support.

For him to make a smooth transition, he has to be able to listen and pay attention to what is expected. And he has to stay calm and open while he gives up one thing and starts the next. It's the staying calm and open part that he doesn't have down yet.

A lot of times, parents can end up bargaining and bribing children to cooperate with a transition. "If you come with me to pick up your sister, I'll give you a candy bar." But this is only a very temporary solution to an ongoing problem. Your child needs to learn to make transitions without a fuss - life is going to require him to make a zillion of them, and he'll cope better if he learns to make them smoothly.

There is a simple and effective technique you can use to help him learn. But it only works if you have been able to trigger self-soothing in Movement 7. In other words, he has to have learned to relax with pressure on the chest. As always, you will use touch to focus his attention and keep him calm and open. This time it will be pressure on the chest.

Let's take an example where he is watching TV and you want him to come to the dinner table. Here's what you do:

1. Make a connection with touch. You sit next to him and without saying anything, place your hands in front of and behind his chest and make a firm, gentle connection.

2. Give the instruction. When you feel that he has noticed you, say: "It's time to come and eat dinner."

3. Repeat and offer help. If he doesn't respond say: "It's time to come and eat dinner; do you need help?"

4. Give physical guidance. If he doesn't respond, keep a steady hold on his chest, and guide him upright saying, "Let's go and eat dinner." You walk next to him, holding his chest until he sees the dinner table and his chair. About then he will be able to complete the transition and get up in his chair.

Okay, there are the steps: make a connection, give the instruction, offer help, give physical guidance.

You'll be surprised how much better it works than just telling him to come to dinner. And there will be no fuss. The reason is that basically he likes dinner, but he doesn't find change easy. Giving his chest pressure before and after gives him extra support that keeps him calm, while he stops doing one thing, and transitions to doing the next. And after a while you'll be able to do the same thing with just a firm, gentle hand on his middle back.

Have fun with that!

Best wishes,

Louisa and Pam

Weekly Log - Week 7

♥ Always start with love

Check each day you do the massage

Sun ___ Mon ___ Tuesday ___ Wed ___ Thu ___ Fri ___ Sat ___

Things You Noticed:

During the Massage

Mv1. Lays down/won't lay down?

Mv2. Back – hums?

Mv3-4. Ears – avoids?

Mv5. Up/up/up – eye contact?

Mv6. Fingers – stroking or pressing?

Mv7. Chest – rubs eyes, yawns, relaxes?

Mv8. Belly – diarrhea/constipation?

Mv9-10. Legs – patting or pressing?

Mv11. Toes – stroking, pressing, bicycle?

Mv12. Soles – avoids?

During the Week

Sleep _____

Bowels _____

Tantrums _____

Affection _____

Eye contact _____

Listening _____

Speaking _____

Other_____

Positive things other people said about your child ...

Your thoughts and feelings about the process ...

Questions you had this week ...

Remember: Look for answers to your questions in the index and the book.

Week 8

Letter to parents – Two extra techniques: The Easy Button, the Face-Me Button

Recommended Reading: *Qigong Massage for Your Child With Autism: A Home Program from Chinese Medicine*, Chapter 7

Dear Parents,

Last week we told you about a special technique to help your child make transitions easier. We hope you've tried it and that it worked well for you.

This week we have two more "bonus" techniques to share with you. The first one helps your child settle down when she is starting to get wound up. The second one helps you get your child's attention.

Like the transition technique we covered last week, these techniques work best with children who have had the benefit of the massage for several weeks or months, as their bodies are more open to touch-cues. Knowing these techniques is a bit like having a button to push to assist your child to turn on certain behaviors. Except you don't push it, you pat it.

We think these extra techniques, which use the same principles as the Qigong massage you're already using, will be very useful to you. And if you discover other techniques, like these parents did, let us know!

The 'Easy Button'

This point is on the top of the head, where we start Movement 1. It is a button to press when your child is winding up and you want her to slow down and go easy. That is why we call it the 'Easy Button'.

One mother told us this story about how she used it. She was waiting for the bus with her son, and he was getting more and more hyper, bouncing up and down. She started patting on the top of his head on that spot, and after a minute he calmed down and stood still by her side until the bus came. She was amazed.

49

Sometimes a medium tapping speed works best, other times a slow pulsing pressure works better. Next time your child starts to wind up, try it and see if it doesn't help her settle down.

You can also use it when your child is toe-walking. Just pat it lightly for a bit, and she will settle down onto her heels.

The 'Face-Me Button'

At the top of his spine, where your child's head meets her neck, is another button we call the 'Face-Me Button'. Refer to the book, Qigong Massage for your Child with Autism, chapter 4, movement 1 to find this spot. You tap into this area during Movement 1 when you loosen up his neck. This button connects directly to the part of the brain that makes her face you when you call her. Facing the person calling their name isn't easy for children with autism – they don't usually answer to their name that way. But it is a skill your child will really need for school, and using this technique together before your child enters school will help her develop that skill.

If she is involved in something, and you want her to face you and pay attention, here is what you do: sit or stand beside her at eye-level, and start patting this spot with the center of your cupped hand over the spot. After you have patted a few times, call her name. You will see, she will turn and face you. You have her attention now, and can talk to her.

At first your child will need the patting on the spot to face the person who is calling their name, but after you have practiced with her enough, she will face you when you call her name without patting first.

Feel free to use these techniques a lot whenever your child needs that extra bit of help settling down or facing you.

All our best,

Louisa and Pam

Weekly Log - Week 8

♥ Always start with love

Check each day you do the massage

Sun ___ Mon ___ Tuesday ___ Wed ___ Thu ___ Fri ___ Sat ___

Things You Noticed:

During the Massage

Mv1. Lays down/won't lay down?

Mv2. Back – hums?

Mv3-4. Ears – avoids?

Mv5. Up/up/up – eye contact?

Mv6. Fingers – stroking or pressing?

Mv7. Chest – rubs eyes, yawns, relaxes?

Mv8. Belly – diarrhea/constipation?

Mv9-10. Legs – patting or pressing?

Mv11. Toes – stroking, pressing, bicycle?

Mv12. Soles – avoids?

During the Week

Sleep _____

Bowels _____

Tantrums _____

Affection _____

Eye contact _____

Listening _____

Speaking _____

Other_____

Positive things other people said about your child ...

Your thoughts and feelings about the process ...

Questions you had this week ...

Remember: Look for answers to your questions in the index and the book.

Week 9

Letter to parents – Solving sleeping problems: Chinese medicine concept – energy flow

Dear Parents,

You already know that Qigong massage is based on Chinese medicine. You don't get very far into Chinese medicine before you bump into the concept of energy flow. In our first book, we weren't sure whether parents would be comfortable learning about energy and how to work with it, and we didn't go into it very much. Since then, we've found that some parents are very interested in this and some aren't. So the information in the next three weekly letters is respectfully offered to those who are. And if this isn't something you're interested in or comfortable with, that's okay, your success with the massage is just as good whether you're interested in energy and Chinese medicine or not.

Either way, you'll definitely want to read these letters because they include some valuable tips for addressing common problems like sleep, listening, language and tantrums.

You already have a common-sense appreciation of energy. You know when you have plenty of energy and when your energy is low. But what might be new to you is how Chinese medicine describes energy flow and energy blocks. If you are wondering what causes an energy block, the list includes toxins, injury, stress, poor diet, infections and irregular sleep.

Energy blocks cause different symptoms and can often be treated with massage. Sleep problems are something many children with autism experience, and it's one example of blocked energy. Let's see how Chinese medicine looks at this problem.

According to Chinese medicine, the natural movement of energy when we go to sleep is down and in. We calm "down", settle "down", and "turn in" for the night.

If energy is blocked and can't flow down, it remains trapped up in the head, and we don't fall asleep. What we say reflects this: "I was 'up' all night," "I couldn't let down."

The neck and shoulders are common areas for energy block – the muscles get tight and knotted and keep the energy trapped in the head. In order for your child to fall asleep, energy has to be able to flow through his neck and shoulders all the way down to his feet. Movements 1 and 2, help it to do that. When your child will lie down during Movements 1 and 2, it means that energy has flowed down and sleep will be better.

That's one kind of sleep problem qigong massage can help. Here's another . . .

What if he falls asleep at night, but wakes up three hours later? Energy flow in the body has not only direction but depth as well. Energy flows down the back of the body through the layers of muscle, not only through the skin. If your child has severe sleep problems, his neck will be more blocked. His neck muscles might be tight all the way to the bone. With the first few massages, you might get the surface to soften. Your child may then fall asleep, but wake up a few hours later. This means the deeper part is still blocked.

The solution is simple. Next time you do the massage, pay more attention to the deep muscles of the neck and shoulders – tap into the nape of his neck with your fingertips until it is soft and relaxed all the way down to the bone. Also pat for a long time on the tops of his shoulders until they are completely loose under your hands. You may have to do this several days in a row. Once you are able to relax the deep part of his neck muscles, the deeper block will have cleared, and he should sleep through the night.

Wishing you many good nights sleep!

Louisa and Pam

Weekly Log - Week 9

♥ Always start with love

Check each day you do the massage

Sun ___ Mon ___ Tuesday ___ Wed ___ Thu ___ Fri ___ Sat ___

Things You Noticed:

During the Massage

Mv1. Lays down/won't lay down?

Mv2. Back – hums?

Mv3-4. Ears – avoids?

Mv5. Up/up/up – eye contact?

Mv6. Fingers – stroking or pressing?

Mv7. Chest – rubs eyes, yawns, relaxes?

Mv8. Belly – diarrhea/constipation?

Mv9-10. Legs – patting or pressing?

Mv11. Toes – stroking, pressing, bicycle?

Mv12. Soles – avoids?

During the Week

Sleep _____

Bowels _____

Tantrums _____

Affection _____

Eye contact _____

Listening _____

Speaking _____

Other_____

Positive things other people said about your child ...

Your thoughts and feelings about the process ...

Questions you had this week ...

Remember: Look for answers to your questions in the index and the book.

Week 10

Letter to parents – Solving listening problems – blocked flow to the ears

Dear Parents,

You will spend a lot of time on your child's ears when you do QST massage, and you will be surprised how much their ears will change. Until now, we have been describing how to work with ears in terms of whether your child wants patting or pressing. Today, we will look at ears from the point of view of blocked energy.

What it amounts to is that you don't want there to be any energy blocks around your child's ears. You don't want any barriers to her feeling and using her ears to listen and learn language. What can you do to help this?

You pay attention to two things that maybe you've never thought of as having anything to do with hearing – the skin and the muscles around the ear. And you use techniques from Chinese medicine that have rarely been seen by Western medicine but that work very well indeed.

In practical terms you start with the skin – with patting and pressing in Movements 3 and 4 until, after a few weeks or months, the surface skin around the ears feels quite comfortable to your touch. But for ears, we need to go a bit deeper and do a bit more. We need to be sure that the neck muscles that attach on the side of the neck just under and behind the ears are completely soft and comfortable, too.

We get to them by tapping into them with our fingertips, and patting on the top of the shoulder at the same time. If there are two of you giving the massage together, one person taps under the ear, and the other pats on the top of the shoulder. If not, you can tap under the ear with one hand and on the top of the shoulder with your other hand. That's fine, too. It speeds up progress to tap both the ear and the shoulder at the same time. That way the whole muscle vibrates and the block shakes loose.

Our very best wishes to all of you.

Louisa and Pam

Weekly Log - Week 10

♥ Always start with love

Check each day you do the massage

Sun ___ Mon ___ Tuesday ___ Wed ___ Thu ___ Fri ___ Sat ___

Things You Noticed:

During the Massage

Mv1. Lays down/won't lay down?

Mv2. Back – hums?

Mv3-4. Ears – avoids?

Mv5. Up/up/up – eye contact?

Mv6. Fingers – stroking or pressing?

Mv7. Chest – rubs eyes, yawns, relaxes?

Mv8. Belly – diarrhea/constipation?

Mv9-10. Legs – patting or pressing?

Mv11. Toes – stroking, pressing, bicycle?

Mv12. Soles – avoids?

During the Week

Sleep _____

Bowels _____

Tantrums _____

Affection _____

Eye contact _____

Listening _____

Speaking _____

Other_____

Positive things other people said about your child ...

Your thoughts and feelings about the process ...

Questions you had this week ...

Remember: Look for answers to your questions in the index and the book.

Week 11

Letter to parents – Solving tantrums - opening up flow to the chest

Dear Parents,

You are getting the idea of how QST massage helps open up circulation to specific areas on the outside of the body, like the back of the body, the ears, and the fingers.

Now let's look at how to open up flow to the inside of the body – the head, chest and belly. In week 9 we talked about energy blocks in the head and what to do about them. This week we'll write about energy blocks in the chest, and next week we'll write about the belly.

When we are stressed and shut down, the chest gets tight. When we are relaxed and open, the chest relaxes.

Inside the chest, around the heart, is a huge network of tiny nerves that respond to a deep out-breath by relaxing the chest so it can breathe in deeply.

When we do Movement 7, we are stimulating those nerves to get a deep relaxation response in a child who has not been used to relaxing. We do the in-and-out pressure of our hands on our child's chest at the speed of the resting heart rate – 60 beats per minute – to remind his body of relaxing to the sound of his mother's heartbeat before he was born.

The ribs are made to be flexible. They expand and contract easily with each deep breath. And it feels good to give them a big hug and squeeze. Think about how much a child's ribs move when they take a deep breath. That is how much you can comfortably move them when you do Movement 7.

And here's an extra bonus – when you do Movement 7 for a full minute, imagine you are delivering the love contained in 60 big hugs!

As you start pressing in and out on each side of the breastbone, at first the ribs may be tight. Stay on areas that are tight, slow down and press gently in and out until they relax. Then continue on down with the movement. Watch your child's face carefully. After a few minutes you will see him yawn or reach up and rub his eyes. Those are signs the relaxation response is turning on! It's also good to remember that the chest is a place we can hold grief, shame and other deep feelings. Later on, your child may release tears from his chest when you work on movement 7. We'll tell you more about how to work with that in Week 14.

And here's the really great news – once you trigger the relaxation response for your child a few times, he will be able to trigger it for himself when he needs it – either to calm down, or to get himself through a transition without having a meltdown.

> *"My daughter is very sensitive and easily over-stimulated.*
> *The massage has really helped her be able to soothe herself.*
> *And the tantrums are basically gone!" - Mom*

Don't be afraid to stay on this area longer and get to know where it is tight. Over time, the chest will be able to move in and out freely. If you see your child's hands come up and cover your own, stay even longer. It means you have really opened up the circulation to his chest, and he wants you to fill it up with good energy.

Good work!

Louisa and Pam

Weekly Log - Week 11

♥ Always start with love

Check each day you do the massage

Sun ___ Mon ___ Tuesday ___ Wed ___ Thu ___ Fri ___ Sat ___

Things You Noticed:

During the Massage

Mv1. Lays down/won't lay down?

Mv2. Back – hums?

Mv3-4. Ears – avoids?

Mv5. Up/up/up – eye contact?

Mv6. Fingers – stroking or pressing?

Mv7. Chest – rubs eyes, yawns, relaxes?

Mv8. Belly – diarrhea/constipation?

Mv9-10. Legs – patting or pressing?

Mv11. Toes – stroking, pressing, bicycle?

Mv12. Soles – avoids?

During the Week

Sleep _____

Bowels _____

Tantrums _____

Affection _____

Eye contact _____

Listening _____

Speaking _____

Other_____

Positive things other people said about your child ...

Your thoughts and feelings about the process ...

Questions you had this week ...

Remember: Look for answers to your questions in the index and the book.

Week 12

Letter to parents – Opening up and strengthening the energy of the belly

Dear Parents,

There is a huge network of nerves in the belly, - one hundred million nerve cells - which help to regulate digestion. All together, they work on turning your child's food into energy and nutrients for growth. Good nutrition is important for all children, but when a child has problems with learning and behavior, it is doubly important.

That is why it is important for your child to eat healthy, home-prepared food. Processed and packaged foods contain man-made chemicals that your child's body cannot turn into brain food. Instead these chemicals hang around and cause problems with learning and behavior.

The physical signs the belly isn't working well are obvious: poor appetite, reflux, diarrhea and constipation. QST massage can do a lot for these problems. You already know how to adjust the massage for diarrhea and constipation, and have probably seen the dark bowel movements that happen when the body expels old waste and starts working better.

If your child has reflux, there are two additional things you need to pay attention to - avoiding ice, and serving food that is warm and cooked. Basically, the stomach is a muscle that mashes the food so that it can be further digested. Ice water cools down the stomach and turns it into a stiff, frozen muscle that doesn't work very well. One of the first things to go wrong is that food doesn't go down - it goes up instead – hence reflux and vomiting. Serving cold, raw food, is another way to create extra work for the stomach. It takes a lot of energy to process raw vegetables – think about how long it takes to cook them.

So, if your child's digestive system is weak, don't feed your child iced, cold or raw food. Take the load off, and provide warm and cooked food and no ice. Yes, they can have fruit, but after the meal, or as a snack - not as the main meal.

Once you get the organs of digestion working smoothly again with diet and massage, there is something deeper in the belly that you will become aware of. The belly is where we hold the emotions of fear and anger. As you are working there, your child may release bubbles of these emotions. Just stay calm, reassure your child by lovingly saying "You're okay," and keep working on the area. The emotions will release and your child will be better off for having let them go. Unless circumstances are unusual, this doesn't happen more than once or twice.

Once your child's belly is relaxed and digestion is working well, you will know your child is getting what they need from their food. Before long, you will be surprised at how much your child grows physically – nutrition turns into real tangible growth.

Also, once the belly is clear using the parent support hands, illustrated in the Qigong at Home Booklet (See Section 1, qigong massage picture storybooks), this will be a nice way to additionally strengthen your child's belly and fill up his reserves.

Best wishes,

Louisa and Pam

Weekly Log - Week 12

♥ Always start with love

Check each day you do the massage

Sun ___ Mon ___ Tuesday ___ Wed ___ Thu ___ Fri ___ Sat ___

Things You Noticed:

During the Massage

Mv1. Lays down/won't lay down?

Mv2. Back – hums?

Mv3-4. Ears – avoids?

Mv5. Up/up/up – eye contact?

Mv6. Fingers – stroking or pressing?

Mv7. Chest – rubs eyes, yawns, relaxes?

Mv8. Belly – diarrhea/constipation?

Mv9-10. Legs – patting or pressing?

Mv11. Toes – stroking, pressing, bicycle?

Mv12. Soles – avoids?

During the Week

Sleep _____

Bowels _____

Tantrums _____

Affection _____

Eye contact _____

Listening _____

Speaking _____

Other_____

Positive things other people said about your child ...

Your thoughts and feelings about the process ...

Questions you had this week ...

Remember: Look for answers to your questions in the index and the book.

Week 13

Letter to parents – QST and other therapies

Dear Parents,

We are often asked about whether QST massage goes well with other autism therapies, and here is our answer. In a nutshell, it goes very well with proven educational therapies, and it does not go with unproven therapies.

QST is like putting glasses on a child who is short-sighted so she can see the teacher giving the lesson, or giving hearing aids to a child who is hard of hearing so she can hear the lesson. QST helps to correct touch problems, but because touch is the mother of all senses, that has beneficial effects on all the senses, both individually and together.

The research shows QST not only normalizes all the sensory responses, it helps the senses work together better. You know this is happening when your child faces you, looks at you, and listens to you all at the same time.

So, if you have your child enrolled in speech therapy, or occupational therapy, or other therapies designed to teach your child skills they need, QST will definitely help your child learn the new skills. Your child will be better able to focus on the teacher, take in the new information, and learn. QST will also help your child to be more aware of themselves and the people around them, so that they can learn more – and learn more naturally – from the experiences you provide for them.

There are several sensory therapies that are widely recommended for autism, e.g. brushing and joint compression, but have little or no research proof of effectiveness for autism. We do not recommend unproven therapies. There are many unproven therapies, some may even be harmful, and all take your valuable time and energy away from things that do work. Stick with what is proven to work!

All the best,

Louisa and Pam

Weekly Log - Week 13

♥ Always start with love

Check each day you do the massage

Sun ___ Mon ___ Tuesday ___ Wed ___ Thu ___ Fri ___ Sat ___

Things You Noticed:

During the Massage

Mv1. Lays down/won't lay down?

Mv2. Back – hums?

Mv3-4. Ears – avoids?

Mv5. Up/up/up – eye contact?

Mv6. Fingers – stroking or pressing?

Mv7. Chest – rubs eyes, yawns, relaxes?

Mv8. Belly – diarrhea/constipation?

Mv9-10. Legs – patting or pressing?

Mv11. Toes – stroking, pressing, bicycle?

Mv12. Soles – avoids?

During the Week

Sleep _____

Bowels _____

Tantrums _____

Affection _____

Eye contact _____

Listening _____

Speaking _____

Other_____

Positive things other people said about your child ...

Your thoughts and feelings about the process ...

Questions you had this week ...

Remember: Look for answers to your questions in the index and the book.

Week 14

Letter to parents – Changes during massage and what they mean

Dear Parent,

So let's see what some of these changes look like. By now you are probably seeing some changes and benefits from the massage, both in terms of your child's behavior and your stress level. But you may not be aware that certain changes in the way your child responds to the massage itself are clues that important improvements are on the horizon. So we thought we'd tell you about a few of these changes so you can look for them. They are like an early warning system that your child's development is about to take off.

Let's see what some of these changes look like.

If your child lies on his belly and puts his head down during the massage, this is a sign that his nervous system is calming down, and he will start sleeping better. If he stays down for the whole massage, you know his sense of touch is getting more normal. And this is super important because when touch gets more normal, the autism gets less severe.

If your child doesn't mind you touching his ears any more and his neck is soft and relaxed, he will start paying more attention to people's voices and understanding more of what you say to him.

If he is looking at you and smiling during movement 5, this means that touch, hearing and vision are coming together for him and he can start to turn towards you, make eye contact and listen. This is the starting point for social development. Pretty soon you'll see him paying attention to other people and starting to interact with them more.

If your child's fingers are more comfortable, then his fine motor skills and speech will start to get better. In fact, in our experience over 90% of children improve in language as a result of Qigong massage. Even more severely autistic, nonverbal children acquire some speech, and those who don't still improve in other areas and parenting stress also goes down.

Yawning or rubbing his eyes during movement 7 means he will be able to calm himself down when he starts getting upset. He'll have fewer meltdowns and the ones he does have will be shorter and milder. And transitions will be easier for him, too.

As his belly gets more normal, he'll be eating more foods and his bowels will be more regular – a growth spurt may be right around the corner.

And as his feet are more comfortable, his gross motor skills will improve.

And the best part about all these changes is that as your child relaxes into the massage you both enjoy this very special time together. You'll discover you can use more nurturing touch with your child outside the massage and you'll feel closer to each other. You'll feel like your batteries are recharged.

And that feels terrific.

All our best,

Louisa and Pam

Weekly Log - Week 14

♥ Always start with love

Check each day you do the massage

Sun ___ Mon ___ Tuesday ___ Wed ___ Thu ___ Fri ___ Sat ___

Things You Noticed:

During the Massage

Mv1. Lays down/won't lay down?

Mv2. Back – hums?

Mv3-4. Ears – avoids?

Mv5. Up/up/up – eye contact?

Mv6. Fingers – stroking or pressing?

Mv7. Chest – rubs eyes, yawns, relaxes?

Mv8. Belly – diarrhea/constipation?

Mv9-10. Legs – patting or pressing?

Mv11. Toes – stroking, pressing, bicycle?

Mv12. Soles – avoids?

During the Week

Sleep _____

Bowels _____

Tantrums _____

Affection _____

Eye contact _____

Listening _____

Speaking _____

Other_____

Positive things other people said about your child ...

Your thoughts and feelings about the process ...

Questions you had this week ...

Remember: Look for answers to your questions in the index and the book.

Week 15

Letter to parents – A child's feelings: emotional release during massage

Dear Parents,

In these letters, we'll be talking about feelings – feelings mothers, fathers and siblings of children with autism experience. Having a family member with autism is challenging. Being a child with autism is challenging, too, and children with autism have many of the same emotions related to their own experience as their family does. And, like any child, they feel their family's pain in addition to their own. But because they typically are unable to express their emotions, they often hold onto them and they can get "stuck" in their bodies. This is really not so different than an adult having chronic headaches or stomach aches as the result of unresolved stress.

Parent touch in qigong massage can open up these emotions in a child and help to finally release them. Don't be surprised if your child suddenly expresses strong emotion during the massage. This most often happens after you have been doing the massage for a few months. It is a very good thing for your child to release this emotion, but it can be very hard for parents to see their child dissolve in sorrowful sobs. So let's talk about what to do if this happens.

The most important thing is to keep doing the part of the massage that you're doing when the emotion comes out – don't stop! This can be very hard to do and probably isn't your natural response. Your instinct will be to stop what you're doing and comfort your child. But what they need is for you to stay calm, slow down and continue the massage when the emotion starts coming out, and stay on that area until the emotion is completely released. Try to be matter of fact and lovingly reassure your child with your voice, "You're okay, you're okay" as they release the emotion. Once it's out, they will be done with it.

"During the massage one day, my son just started sobbing. If I hadn't been warned about this I definitely would have stopped

right then! But I kept doing what I was doing and the sobbing stopped just as quickly as it had started. He didn't seem to really even notice he had been sobbing. It felt like something deep inside that needed to come out came out."

Some emotions are more common with specific movements of the massage. For example, during movement 7 children may release sorrow or grief, breaking out into heart-wrenching sobs – as we've said, you keep doing Movement 7. During movement 8, fear or shock, or even anger sometimes comes out. You may see the feeling start to bubble up, and if you stop or get alarmed, it will not come out. Keep doing the movement, stay calm, reassure your child and the emotion will release quickly and not return. Once the emotion is out, just continue on with the rest of the massage as usual.

Emotion coming out is a sign that the areas that have been holding these emotions are opening up and healing. It's a wonderful sign that the massage is working. And it is pretty likely that you'll see some profound change in your child's behavior following such an emotional release. For example, if she is normally tense, she may become much more relaxed and open.

Not all children have emotional releases during qigong massage, but many do. So anticipating that it can happen and knowing what to do will help you be prepared to respond in the best way for your child.

Best wishes,

Louisa and Pam

Weekly Log - Week 15

♥ Always start with love

Check each day you do the massage

Sun ___ Mon ___ Tuesday ___ Wed ___ Thu ___ Fri ___ Sat ___

Things You Noticed:

During the Massage

Mv1. Lays down/won't lay down?

Mv2. Back – hums?

Mv3-4. Ears – avoids?

Mv5. Up/up/up – eye contact?

Mv6. Fingers – stroking or pressing?

Mv7. Chest – rubs eyes, yawns, relaxes?

Mv8. Belly – diarrhea/constipation?

Mv9-10. Legs – patting or pressing?

Mv11. Toes – stroking, pressing, bicycle?

Mv12. Soles – avoids?

During the Week

Sleep _____

Bowels _____

Tantrums _____

Affection _____

Eye contact _____

Listening _____

Speaking _____

Other_____

Positive things other people said about your child ...

Your thoughts and feelings about the process ...

Questions you had this week ...

Remember: Look for answers to your questions in the index and the book.

70

Week 16

Letter to parents – Still hyper? Food makes a difference

Recommended Reading: *Qigong Massage for Your Child With Autism: A Home Program from Chinese Medicine*, Chapters 9 and 10

Dear parents,

By week 10, you will be noticing some changes. But if the changes seem to be less than you expected, it's time to think carefully about diet. A study done in England with several thousand children reported that red dye in food caused hyperactive behavior. Nowadays, packaged foods for children are highly processed and contain a lot of food coloring, sugar and other additives.

Children with autism are slower to process chemical additives than their typically developing peers, and the effects of such toxins are stronger and last longer in their bodies than their peers.

We're thinking of one little girl with high functioning autism that would talk non-stop. She has almost no awareness of how her behavior affected other children, and there were lots of complaints from her teacher about non-stop talking and disrupting classroom activities. Other children didn't want to be her friend. She ate an almost constant diet of pop, chips, candy and fast food.

Her Mom decided to take all the junk out of her diet. She switched the whole family over to whole foods and offered them water to drink. No more pop, no more chips, no more candy. It was homemade meals and fruit for snacks.

The change in her daughter was like day and night. She calmed down and started listening. She stopped talking all the time. And the reports from school came back better right away.

This is a pretty extreme example, but it does illustrate the point. So if your child is hyper, take a close look at the diet, and try taking out the sugar, food coloring and processed food for a few weeks. You might be very pleased with what happens, and see faster progress with massage.

Best wishes, Louisa and Pam

Weekly Log - Week 16

♥ Always start with love

Check each day you do the massage

Sun ___ Mon ___ Tuesday ___ Wed ___ Thu ___ Fri ___ Sat ___

Things You Noticed:

During the Massage

Mv1. Lays down/won't lay down?

Mv2. Back – hums?

Mv3-4. Ears – avoids?

Mv5. Up/up/up – eye contact?

Mv6. Fingers – stroking or pressing?

Mv7. Chest – rubs eyes, yawns, relaxes?

Mv8. Belly – diarrhea/constipation?

Mv9-10. Legs – patting or pressing?

Mv11. Toes – stroking, pressing, bicycle?

Mv12. Soles – avoids?

During the Week

Sleep _____

Bowels _____

Tantrums _____

Affection _____

Eye contact _____

Listening _____

Speaking _____

Other_____

Positive things other people said about your child ...

Your thoughts and feelings about the process ...

Questions you had this week ...

Remember: Look for answers to your questions in the index and the book.

Week 17

Letter to parents – A simple thing to do to stop aggressive behavior

Dear parents,

Children with autism can have all sorts of aggressive behaviors – pinching, hitting, kicking, biting and even spitting. The behaviors are usually triggered really fast, sometimes with only a one- or two-second warning to tell you they are coming.

There is a very simple reason for this. And it is not that your child is an aggressive person. It's because the part of the brain called the autonomic nervous system is tipped towards fight and flight, and your child hasn't yet learned how to deal with pain, threat or frustration appropriately.

The brain has two parts that are responsible for survival. The technical terms are the sympathetic nervous system and the parasympathetic nervous system. The first helps your child survive by self-defense ("fight and flight") and the second helps your child survive by getting along with others and behaving appropriately ("relax and relate").

In the young child, "fight-mode" and the aggressive behavior that goes with it is commonly triggered by one of three things: 1) touch which is painful; 2) someone coming into the child's personal space too quickly, or taking something which belongs to the child; or 3) the child getting frustrated.

In contrast, "relax-and-relate-mode" is triggered by one thing – reassuring parent touch. Sound familiar? We are talking about the same part of the brain that is responsible for the self-regulation abilities that we have been exploring – sleep, self-soothing, attention, etc. But it has one more extremely important function – it dials down the "fight and flight" part of the brain. And it makes your child receptive to learning appropriate behavior.

Children aren't born knowing appropriate behavior; they have to learn it from their parents. When a child is being aggressive, parents have to stop the behavior, get him out of "fight-mode" and into a more receptive state, and teach him how to behave appropriately.

When you see aggressive behavior, you will want to act in the moment to stop it, and you will need to remain calm. What we are going to suggest won't work if you do it five or ten minutes later, and it won't work if you get upset.

Here is what you do. If your child has pinched or hit, you reach out and firmly but gently squeeze the hand that pinched or hit and say in a calm, firm voice, "No hitting/pinching – gentle hands." It will surprise your child. Firm pressure will focus her awareness on her body and help to switch her brain over into "receptive-mode." She will hear you. Continue firm pressure until you feel her hands relax.

If you sense your child is going to kick, take both feet firmly in your hands, squeeze and say, "No kicking – gentle feet." If he is lying down, put gentle pressure above both knees and say the same thing. Continue until he relaxes his legs.

If the behavior is biting or spitting, you can firmly grasp both shoulders and press, and then firmly but gently press down the arms to the hands, while saying, "No biting/spitting – gentle." Repeat this several times, holding his hands firmly in yours.

Usually the behavior stops immediately. If your child is verbal, you can talk with him about what happened and encourage him to use his words instead. Depending on the child, you can also say, "When we are frustrated, we use our words." If he is non-verbal, it is often enough to just stop the behavior.

You may need to repeat this in the future when the behavior recurs, but often the frequency of the behavior drops quickly. It's a good way to help your child learn appropriate behavior.

Once you get the hang of it, we think it will work well for you.

Best of luck,

Louisa and Pam

Weekly Log - Week 17

♥ Always start with love

Check each day you do the massage

Sun ___ Mon ___ Tuesday ___ Wed ___ Thu ___ Fri ___ Sat ___

Things You Noticed:

During the Massage

Mv1. Lays down/won't lay down?

Mv2. Back – hums?

Mv3-4. Ears – avoids?

Mv5. Up/up/up – eye contact?

Mv6. Fingers – stroking or pressing?

Mv7. Chest – rubs eyes, yawns, relaxes?

Mv8. Belly – diarrhea/constipation?

Mv9-10. Legs – patting or pressing?

Mv11. Toes – stroking, pressing, bicycle?

Mv12. Soles – avoids?

During the Week

Sleep _____

Bowels _____

Tantrums _____

Affection _____

Eye contact _____

Listening _____

Speaking _____

Other_____

Positive things other people said about your child ...

Your thoughts and feelings about the process ...

Questions you had this week ...

Remember: Look for answers to your questions in the index and the book.

Week 18

Letter to parents – The "dog days" of a year-long intervention

Dear Parents,

In some ways these can be the "dog days" of doing Qigong massage with your child. The reason you worked so hard to get the massage into your daily family routine is so it would just be a part of how you do things when the going got a little tough. Not all of you will experience these "dog days," but some of you will, so we thought it was important to let you know this and to help you keep going through it.

"Dog days" can look and feel different to different families depending on your experience with the massage to this point. So we thought we'd describe a couple ways this might happen for you and make a few suggestions that might help you through it.

The first few months of massage can be very exciting. You are growing in confidence, your child is enjoying the massage, you're seeing some really exciting improvements, and all of this is very motivating. It keeps you doing the massage every day. Progress can slow down some now that the big issues are resolving and your child is doing better. Parents who let up on the massage now learn very quickly how important it is to continue with it when their child regresses all of a sudden and they realize they have been slipping a bit on their daily massages. That's usually enough to get through the "dog days." We can sometimes even forget a little bit what it was like before. It helps to remember, "Oh, yeah, he used to not go to sleep until 2:00am, now he's falling asleep at 9:00pm." Or to realize, "Wow, he hasn't had a meltdown in weeks." Reviewing your earlier Weekly Logs will remind you how far you've come and reenergize your commitment.

For some of you, your first few months of massage have been a little more challenging. Maybe your child couldn't lie down for the massage and you've had to chase him around and give it in stages throughout the day. Maybe he is still not paying attention when you call his name. Maybe the meltdowns are still happening on a regular basis. Maybe you're beginning to doubt that the massage is going to work for you and your child. This is another way "dog days" can look – tired, confused, frustrated. If this is you, take heart – if you are doing the massage correctly, doing it every day and tuning in to your child's responses and changing from patting to pressing as needed, you will get results. Children are all different, and some will make smaller improvements more slowly, but all will progress. Again, it helps to remember the small changes – that's why we encourage you to write them down on your Weekly Log so you can look back and see the small steps.

Finally, some of you may even be completely overwhelmed right now. If you're not sure you're doing this right, if you're confused about your child's responses and what they mean and how to adapt the massage, or if you're just not seeing much progress, maybe you need some help. You can get coaching and support from a QST therapist through the Qigong Sensory Training Institute at qsti.org. So, reach out and get some help – and don't give up.

The main point is, if you are experiencing the "dog days," shake things up a little. Recommit to doing the massage every day, get another family member to do it with you, write in your Weekly Log every week to keep yourself motivated, journal, make a list of all the small improvements you've seen in your child, and get help and support if you need it.

This is where the rubber really meets the road. We know you can keep going. After all, you've come a long way already.

All our best,

Louisa and Pam

Weekly Log - Week 18

♥ Always start with love

Check each day you do the massage

Sun ___ Mon ___ Tuesday ___ Wed ___ Thu ___ Fri ___ Sat ___

Things You Noticed:

During the Massage

Mv1. Lays down/won't lay down?

Mv2. Back – hums?

Mv3-4. Ears – avoids?

Mv5. Up/up/up – eye contact?

Mv6. Fingers – stroking or pressing?

Mv7. Chest – rubs eyes, yawns, relaxes?

Mv8. Belly – diarrhea/constipation?

Mv9-10. Legs – patting or pressing?

Mv11. Toes – stroking, pressing, bicycle?

Mv12. Soles – avoids?

During the Week

Sleep _____

Bowels _____

Tantrums _____

Affection _____

Eye contact _____

Listening _____

Speaking _____

Other_____

Positive things other people said about your child ...

Your thoughts and feelings about the process ...

Questions you had this week ...

Remember: Look for answers to your questions in the index and the book.

Week 19

Letter to parents – Parenting skills for "The Terrible Twos"

Dear Parents,

Most parents who have experienced their child losing skills are terrified of regressions because they are afraid of losing their child again. Some things can look like a regression – like when your child is suddenly refusing to cooperate and saying "No!" but this is absolutely not a regression. It is a huge sign of progress. It's called the Terrible Twos. This is what it can look like . . .

This stage of development naturally happens around two years of age. Even though your child might be five or six years old, chances are she has never gone through it. It has come about now as a result of all your hard work. Her skin is no longer a patchwork of contradictory feelings of discomfort and numbness. Now her brain can read her whole skin as a single unified message of where her body is. What she understands from that, amazingly, is that she is her own person.

Now, she will take great pleasure in saying "No!" And of course, like everything else, once she learns she can say "No" she wants to practice it. We once counted 17 "No's" during a single conversation with a child. It takes some effort to remember that this is a good sign of progress! Now you need to shift your parenting style and offer your child choices. If she says "No" to putting her sweater on, offer her a choice – does she want to put her sweater on herself, or does she want you to help her? She will always make the choice. That is what she wants – to have a say in what happens. And you can let her have a say. It doesn't mean she has control, but there is almost always something about the situation where she can have a choice.

Children will also come out with the most amazing things when they become aware of themselves as their own person. Like one little boy who used to talk almost constantly about a cartoon character – one day, out of the blue, told his mother, "I want to be a child. I don't want to be a grown-up." Then he went right back to saying "No!"

When you start hearing "No!" a lot, your parenting style needs to shift to parenting a toddler. This stage is about learning to deal with having more freedom and staying safe –it's about choices, rules and limits. Your child needs to learn when he has the freedom to make choices and when he has to follow the rules. Offer your child choices whenever it is appropriate, and set firm consistent limits and hold to them when you need to. He will learn that he has some freedom and that you will keep him safe. And don't be flummoxed by having to teach two-year-old skills to a five year old! Be encouraged that they will learn these skills faster at five than they would have at two.

When children get QST massage, they start developing more normally again. They go back and pick up skills that they missed out on earlier. This is what we call "catch-up" development. The Terrible Twos don't usually last as long in older children as they would in a typical two-year-old; maybe it will take him only a few weeks to understand the difference between something he has a choice about and something that is not his decision. And he'll learn to trust you to give him the freedom he can handle and keep him safe the rest of the time. And then he'll be on to the next phase.

Sometimes parents have been so traumatized by their child's tantrums that they are afraid to set limits with their child and stick to them. Don't be. Keep doing the massage; he won't slip back. He has been learning to self-soothe and now he has shorter and milder tantrums. He is ready to learn to accept rules and limits.

Congratulations! If your child has hit this phase, his development is progressing.

Good work!

Louisa and Pam

Weekly Log - Week 19

♥ Always start with love

Check each day you do the massage

Sun ___ Mon ___ Tuesday ___ Wed ___ Thu ___ Fri ___ Sat ___

Things You Noticed:

During the Massage

Mv1. Lays down/won't lay down?

Mv2. Back – hums?

Mv3-4. Ears – avoids?

Mv5. Up/up/up – eye contact?

Mv6. Fingers – stroking or pressing?

Mv7. Chest – rubs eyes, yawns, relaxes?

Mv8. Belly – diarrhea/constipation?

Mv9-10. Legs – patting or pressing?

Mv11. Toes – stroking, pressing, bicycle?

Mv12. Soles – avoids?

During the Week

Sleep _____

Bowels _____

Tantrums _____

Affection _____

Eye contact _____

Listening _____

Speaking _____

Other_____

Positive things other people said about your child ...

Your thoughts and feelings about the process ...

Questions you had this week ...

Remember: Look for answers to your questions in the index and the book.

Week 20

Letter to parents – Parenting skills for "The Controlling Fours"

Dear Parents,

Last week we talked about the Terrible Twos as a sign of progress from qigong massage. We said that it's best dealt with by setting appropriate rules and limits, but that this can be hard for some parents who have been traumatized by their child's tantrums. This week we're going to talk about another pretty common situation some families find themselves in, which is related to difficulties parents have in parenting the Terrible Twos, and what parents can do about it.

Some children with high functioning autism start QST massage stuck in what we call "The Controlling Fours." This phase is a tough one to live with. But it is not hard to move on from.

Here is how it looks: the child makes rules for the family, and the family obeys. The child doesn't want to go out to breakfast, and the family doesn't go out to breakfast. The child doesn't want the mother to pay attention to anyone else, and the mother doesn't.

In other words, the child hasn't learned the main lesson of the Terrible Twos, which is that parents can be counted on to set boundaries (rules and limits) for what is safe and appropriate behavior. If the parents haven't been able to do this, the child will try to take control of the parents and feel safe that way. But that never works, and nobody is happy.

There is only one way out of this situation: take back control. Let your child know that even though he might want to control other people, he can't; he can only control himself. Let him know that it is your job as his parent to keep him safe, and that means you will set rules and limits, and that you'll enforce them. And then get through the adjustment period where he tests your resolve to be consistent. Be prepared for a few tantrums. Use timeouts and be very consistent. This transition period often doesn't take more than a few days if both parents are together on how they are handling it.

The whole family will breathe a sigh of relief when this stage is behind you.

Good job!

Louisa and Pam

Weekly Log - Week 20

♥ Always start with love

Check each day you do the massage

Sun ___ Mon ___ Tuesday ___ Wed ___ Thu ___ Fri ___ Sat ___

Things You Noticed:

During the Massage

Mv1. Lays down/won't lay down?

Mv2. Back – hums?

Mv3-4. Ears – avoids?

Mv5. Up/up/up – eye contact?

Mv6. Fingers – stroking or pressing?

Mv7. Chest – rubs eyes, yawns, relaxes?

Mv8. Belly – diarrhea/constipation?

Mv9-10. Legs – patting or pressing?

Mv11. Toes – stroking, pressing, bicycle?

Mv12. Soles – avoids?

During the Week

Sleep _____

Bowels _____

Tantrums _____

Affection _____

Eye contact _____

Listening _____

Speaking _____

Other _____

Positive things other people said about your child ...

Your thoughts and feelings about the process ...

Questions you had this week ...

Remember: Look for answers to your questions in the index and the book.

Week 21
Letter to parents – What to do about regression

Dear Parent,

The last couple of weeks we've been talking about things that might look like regression – the Terrible Two's and the Controlling Four's – but are actually signs of progress. Because their autism got in the way, our children didn't go through these stages when they were that age, so they go through them later as the result of Qigong massage.

This week we want to talk a little more about regression. As parents of children with autism, we can get especially alarmed by signs of regression because we remember the pain of our child's regression into autism.

All children have regressions. Regressions simply mean a child is having trouble dealing with her life at that moment. Depending on the cause, they can be small or big, last a few days or a few weeks. Small regressions can happen if a child gets too tired, hungry or stressed. In these cases, a little rest, a good meal, or a little break and downtime and a good night's sleep are usually all that's needed. Bigger regressions happen in response to life's bigger changes and losses, and let us know that our child needs more ongoing emotional support and downtime to regroup and integrate. As long as parents catch on to the reasons for the regression and provide the extra support and down time needed, the regressions don't need to get out of hand.

It also helps to remember that these types of regressions that all children have are temporary. And you're especially lucky, because there are some specific things you can do with Qigong that help with regressions! So, let's take a look at some more common signs you might see as regression and how you can use Qigong to help.

Illness: Regressions are especially common after an illness or injury, as the child struggles to deal with the changes in their body. Be patient. You may have to change your qigong technique, patting more to clear out the toxins from the illness or the blocked circulation from the injury and then pressing to strengthen again. So, just continue the massage and in a few days – or a few weeks in some cases – your child will recover from the illness and the regression it caused. You could even give the massage more than once a day to support her in her recovery.

Skin sensitivity: Some children, who previously have not felt their skin very much, don't know when they are hurt or notice when you touch them, may all of a sudden become completely overwhelmed by touch. Their skin is making the transition from under-sensitive to over-sensitive; suddenly they're taking in a lot more sensory information, and it can be overwhelming. This is not a regression, it is a sign of progress that Qigong massage is helping restore normal sensation to the skin! And it is temporary; your child will get used to the new sensations and adjust to them over time. Not all children experience this, of course, but some do and typically between the second and fourth months of massage. If this happens, switch to pressing/filling on all the movements, do lots of movement 7 and consider increasing the massage to twice a day. In a few weeks, your child will get comfortable and her sensory reactivity will go back to normal.

Toxins: Regression can also be the result of toxins from something a child eats (food, red dye, MSG, etc.) or exposure to fumes from magic markers, solvents or other chemicals. It is relatively easy to clean up the diet, remove junk food, eliminate red dye and remove toxins from the home when you think this could be a reason for regressive behavior – and the results can be dramatic improvement. Doing the massage twice a day will also help move these toxins out of your child's body and toxic reactions will pass within a few days once the offending substance is removed.

Emotions: Qigong massage helps children become more aware of themselves and their emotions. Now they have to process some difficult emotions they haven't previously been in touch with. This can cause emotional reactions that we're not used to in our children. Again, this isn't a regression, but a sign of progress. Give your child space, emotional support and continue the whole massage, attuning carefully to where she needs more nurturing or strengthening (pressing) and where she needs help clearing out (patting). This can be a challenging few weeks, but keep up the massage and she will work through the backlog of emotion and be much better in touch with, and able to process, emotion as it comes up.

Growth spurt: Sometimes just before or after a big growth spurt, the child will have a little regression. Again, you can increase the massage to twice a day and be sure to spend lots of time on movement 7 for extra support. Your child will often need more pressing during that time.

Temporary ups and downs of life: If after considering this list of possible causes of regression you still don't know why your child is showing regressive symptoms, you can assume that she is stressed in some way. Just keep doing the massage and do lots of movement 7 – it will help her to calm down and process the stress.

Bigger life changes: Here your child with autism is no different than any other child. He can regress in response to all the usual life changes and losses that would cause any young child to regress – trouble in school, change to a new school or a new class, changes at home, illness in the family, loss of a care-giver, etc. As in all these other cases, you'll want to be particularly dedicated to continuing the daily massage. It will calm him down and support him while he processes the change or loss. It will calm you down, too, and give you some healing intimate time with your child. Also make sure he is sleeping enough and eating well, which applies to parents, too!

So, if you do encounter some of these signs of regression, you have some specific Qigong massage tools to help your child – and you – move through the regression successfully.

Best wishes,

Louisa and Pam

Weekly Log - Week 21

♥ Always start with love

Check each day you do the massage

Sun ___ Mon ___ Tuesday ___ Wed ___ Thu ___ Fri ___ Sat ___

Things You Noticed:

During the Massage

Mv1. Lays down/won't lay down?

Mv2. Back – hums?

Mv3-4. Ears – avoids?

Mv5. Up/up/up – eye contact?

Mv6. Fingers – stroking or pressing?

Mv7. Chest – rubs eyes, yawns, relaxes?

Mv8. Belly – diarrhea/constipation?

Mv9-10. Legs – patting or pressing?

Mv11. Toes – stroking, pressing, bicycle?

Mv12. Soles – avoids?

During the Week

Sleep _____

Bowels _____

Tantrums _____

Affection _____

Eye contact _____

Listening _____

Speaking _____

Other_____

Positive things other people said about your child …

Your thoughts and feelings about the process …

Questions you had this week …

Remember: Look for answers to your questions in the index and the book.

Week 22
Letter to parents – Mid-year testing

Dear Parent,

Back at the beginning of your adventure with Qigong massage, we said there were a lot of ways to measure progress. You've been getting a gut sense of how the massage has helped your child, and in another month you'll revisit the goals you set for the massage and see how many have been reached. We hope you also completed the two simple tests we offered at the beginning – the Autism Touch/Pain Checklist and the Autism Parenting Stress Index – because this is the measure of progress we're going to have you work with this week.

You might remember that the Autism Touch/Pain Checklist measures how severe your child's touch/pain problems were and the Autism Parenting Stress index evaluates how challenging it is to parent your child. We're going to have you complete these same tests again now and see how the scores have changed since you started the massage six months ago. You know by watching your child that he has improved over the last six months. And these scores are going to show exactly how much he has improved. This is exactly what scientists do to "prove" that something works – or doesn't work. And it's how therapists track children's progress. And you can use the same approach as a parent.

First complete the two simple tests, below. Then we'll tell you how to use the information.

Autism Touch/Pain Checklist

Circle the response for each item that most accurately describes your child.

Touch/Pain	Often	Sometimes	Rarely	Never
• Does not cry tears when hurt	3	2	1	0
• Doesn't notice if the diaper is wet or dirty	3	2	1	0
• Face washing is difficult	3	2	1	0

• Haircuts are difficult	3	2	1	0
• Refuses to wear a hat	3	2	1	0
• Prefers to wear a hat	3	2	1	0
• Cutting fingernails is difficult	3	2	1	0
• Prefers to wear one or two gloves	3	2	1	0
• Avoids wearing gloves	3	2	1	0
• Cutting toenails is difficult	3	2	1	0
• Will only wear certain footwear (e.g. soft shoes, no socks)	3	2	1	0
• Prefers to wear the same clothes day after day	3	2	1	0
• Will only wear certain clothes (e.g. no elastic, no tags, only short pants)	3	2	1	0
• Cries tears when falls, scrapes skin or gets hurt (scale is reversed on purpose)	0	1	2	3
• Head bangs on a hard surface	3	2	1	0
• Head bangs on a soft surface	3	2	1	0
Add up the scores in each column:	___	___	___	___

Add up the total score: _____

The Autism Parenting Stress Index

Please rate the following aspects of your child's health **according to how much stress it causes you and/or your family** by placing an X in the box that best describes your situation.	**Not stressful**	**Sometimes creates stress**	**Often creates stress**	**Very stressful on a daily basis**	**So stressful at times I feel I cannot cope**
Your child's ability to communicate					
Tantrums/meltdowns					
Aggressive behavior (siblings, peers)					
Self-injurious behavior					
Difficulty making transitions from one activity to another					
Sleep problems					
Your child's diet					
Bowel problems (diarrhea, constipation)					
Potty training					
Not feeling close to your child					
Concern for the future of your child being accepted by others					
Concern for the future of your child living independently					

Subtotal: _____   _____   _____   _____   _____

Total: _____

Ok, great! Now let's compare these scores with the scores from the same tests you completed back at the beginning. Fill in the blanks, below:

First Autism Touch/Pain Checklist Total Score: _____

Today's Autism Touch/Pain Checklist Total Score: _____

First Autism Parenting Index Total Score: _____

Today's Autism Parenting Index Total Score: _____

What did you find? Did the scores go down? Depending on how severe your child's autism was to begin with, the scores may have come down a lot or a little. But they probably did come down. So, how does this match what you're seeing in your child?

Scores coming down on the Touch/Pain Checklist

This mean that your child's problems with touch are improving. So the areas of his body that were over-sensitive to touch are calming down, and areas that he didn't feel are awakening, and he is now feeling them. Touch is becoming more normal. Maybe it's a little easier to cut his nails and hair now. Or maybe he'll eat some foods with different textures now. And when he falls down and gets hurt, he cries now. Maybe he even has a dry diaper sometimes or is starting to sit on the potty! The massage has brought an awareness of your child's body and now you can begin to see the independent little person coming out.

> "QST not only handed me the key, but swung the door wide open to the little boy locked away inside and let him out. I never dreamed he'd emerge so tuned in, so vocal, so inquisitive, so loving, so aware and so happy." - Mom, 4 year old boy

Remember when we said at the beginning that problems with touch get in the way of social development in autism, and that parent touch is central to social learning? You've been attuning your touch to your child's body with massage for months now, so you may be able to touch your child a bit more, to comfort him when he cries, use touch to help transitions, or maybe he'll now sit on your lap when you read to him. This is the foundation for social learning – connecting with you, others in the family, and eventually peers.

Scores coming down on the Autism Parenting Stress Index

This means that parenting your child is less stressful than it was before you began the massage. You probably don't need these scores to tell you that! And if these scores did not go down, we've found it's often because parents are more aware of what to look for, more focused on making progress. It's like one parent said, "I didn't even know I should be worried about these things – it's just the way things were. Now I'm stressing about potty training because we're actually working on potty training! Before I didn't even know it was possible, so why stress about it?"

In another six months, at the end of the year of Qigong massage, you'll complete these same tests again and see how much more progress you've made. Some children progress quickly at the beginning and more slowly as the year goes along. Others progress more slowly and first and then pick up later. This is just a mid-year check up. You'll want to keep the massage going every day to see what you can accomplish in another six months!

And remember, if you're feeling uncertain or want to talk with a QST therapist, you can access this support from the Qigong Sensory Training Institute website at qsti.org.

All our best,

Louisa and Pam

Weekly Log - Week 22

♥ Always start with love

Check each day you do the massage

Sun ___ Mon ___ Tuesday ___ Wed ___ Thu ___ Fri ___ Sat ___

Things You Noticed:

During the Massage

Mv1. Lays down/won't lay down?

Mv2. Back – hums?

Mv3-4. Ears – avoids?

Mv5. Up/up/up – eye contact?

Mv6. Fingers – stroking or pressing?

Mv7. Chest – rubs eyes, yawns, relaxes?

Mv8. Belly – diarrhea/constipation?

Mv9-10. Legs – patting or pressing?

Mv11. Toes – stroking, pressing, bicycle?

Mv12. Soles – avoids?

During the Week

Sleep _____

Bowels _____

Tantrums _____

Affection _____

Eye contact _____

Listening _____

Speaking _____

Other_____

Positive things other people said about your child ...

Your thoughts and feelings about the process ...

Questions you had this week ...

Remember: Look for answers to your questions in the index and the book.

Week 23

Letter to parents – Checking in on your goals

Dear Parent,

This week we're going to talk about another way of measuring progress with Qigong massage. At the beginning of your adventure with Qigong massage, you wrote down three things you most wanted the massage to change, and we told you that you'd come back to them in six months and see what has been accomplished. And, here we are!

Look back to the beginning on this workbook and find your three goals. Rewrite your goals here:

1.

2.

3.

Do you see any of the changes you wanted to see when you started the massage? Have any of these things gotten even a little bit easier? Do you see some small steps toward these goals?

Write down one thing you've noticed that shows that the massage is helping each of the three things you wanted the massage to change.

1.

2.

3.

Could you do it? If so, that's terrific! If you're not so sure, hang in there. You're only half way through the year. Keep these goals in mind and watch for small changes that mean the goals are within reach. And remember to celebrate them when you see them.

We're celebrating with you. Keep up the good work.

All our best,

Louisa and Pam

Weekly Log - Week 23

♥ Always start with love

Check each day you do the massage

Sun ___ Mon ___ Tuesday ___ Wed ___ Thu ___ Fri ___ Sat ___

Things You Noticed:

During the Massage

Mv1. Lays down/won't lay down?

Mv2. Back – hums?

Mv3-4. Ears – avoids?

Mv5. Up/up/up – eye contact?

Mv6. Fingers – stroking or pressing?

Mv7. Chest – rubs eyes, yawns, relaxes?

Mv8. Belly – diarrhea/constipation?

Mv9-10. Legs – patting or pressing?

Mv11. Toes – stroking, pressing, bicycle?

Mv12. Soles – avoids?

During the Week

Sleep _____

Bowels _____

Tantrums _____

Affection _____

Eye contact _____

Listening _____

Speaking _____

Other_____

Positive things other people said about your child ...

Your thoughts and feelings about the process ...

Questions you had this week ...

Remember: Look for answers to your questions in the index and the book.

Week 24

Letter to parents – Doing the massage 6-7 days a week vs. 3-4 days a week in the second half of the year

Dear Parents,

It is really important to keep doing the massage 6-7 days a week in order to keep advancing the progress of your child during the first year of QST massage. Most parents don't have too much trouble doing that for the first six months because their children's improvements are so obvious and satisfying. For the second half of year, when children tend to settle down into a less dramatic pattern of growth, that may not be the case. In our research studies, we tracked the results in the first and second half of the year for parents who did the massage 6-7 days a week and for those who dropped back to 3-4 days a week, and we found a big difference!

In the second half of the year, parents who continued the massage 6-7 days a week could expect the same amount of new developmental skills as they saw in the first half of the year. So, for example, if their child improved 20% in language by mid-year, they could go to 40% by the end of the year. But the parents who dropped the frequency of massage to 3-4 days a week in the second half of the year did not get the same results. Their children kept the gains they had made in the first half of the year, but did not keep gaining skills at the same rate as those who got the massage every day. It was like they moved from catch-up mode to maintenance mode.

Medicines wear off and need to be given regularly. Massage is the most organizing, relaxing and energizing medicine we have. It boosts your child's nervous system in the direction of growth every single day. Your child's nervous system has been in a pattern of delayed growth for several years. If you want to change an established pattern, you need to give the daily treatment for at least half as long as the pattern has been in place. So if your child regressed into autism 3 years ago and you want to shift him onto a better path and keep him improving, you might plan to give the massage for 1 ½ years. If he only regressed 2 years ago, you could plan for daily massage for one year.

Having said that, there are exceptions. The research showed that some children, specifically the higher-functioning ones, did continue to make good progress in the second half of the year with massage 3-4 days a week. So observe closely, know what the research says, know there are always exceptions, and make your decision based on your child. Continuing daily massage is never a bad idea!

All our best,

Louisa and Pam

Weekly Log - Week 24

♥ Always start with love

Check each day you do the massage

Sun ___ Mon ___ Tuesday ___ Wed ___ Thu ___ Fri ___ Sat ___

Things You Noticed:

During the Massage

Mv1. Lays down/won't lay down?

Mv2. Back – hums?

Mv3-4. Ears – avoids?

Mv5. Up/up/up – eye contact?

Mv6. Fingers – stroking or pressing?

Mv7. Chest – rubs eyes, yawns, relaxes?

Mv8. Belly – diarrhea/constipation?

Mv9-10. Legs – patting or pressing?

Mv11. Toes – stroking, pressing, bicycle?

Mv12. Soles – avoids?

During the Week

Sleep _____

Bowels _____

Tantrums _____

Affection _____

Eye contact _____

Listening _____

Speaking _____

Other_____

Positive things other people said about your child ...

Your thoughts and feelings about the process ...

Questions you had this week ...

Remember: Look for answers to your questions in the index and the book.

Week 25

Letter to parents – A skeptical parent comes to believe

Dear Parents,

I first heard about QST from my son's OT a few months after he started school, he had just turned six. Initially I was skeptical, it sounded like one of those mystic energy healing things I definitely didn't believe in. Then the OT showed me some of the scientific studies that found QST was effective and I was intrigued.

By the time of our next OT meeting a week later, I had bought a copy of the book and read it and had copies of all the studies that had been published. I was starting to be convinced. The scientific studies made all the difference to me.

At that time my son was having a very difficult time adjusting to school, he was hitting the staff and I was worried he would be thrown out of school. My house was very clean though as I couldn't sleep and was up most nights cleaning! He had many sensory challenges - hypersensitive to light, sound and some touch (he wouldn't wear socks). He also didn't like it when other children cried, including babies. At the park, we had to rush to be near him if a child cried as there was a risk of him hitting the child in an effort to stop the crying. A few times we were not fast enough and he did hit children at the beach, park and school.

He was not sleeping well, would sometimes take a long time to fall asleep or he would wake up in the middle of the night and not be able to go back to sleep. I always heard him so I didn't sleep much either. He would have some spectacular tantrums that could last for what seemed like forever. I used to call him my Ferrari because he could go from 0-60 in a few seconds. Food was another challenge, he was a very fussy eater.

When I started using QST, to be honest I wasn't expecting much. I decided I would commit to doing the massage faithfully for the five months indicated in the studies I'd read, and I was going to evaluate it then.

Around Christmas my son's class went to the nearby shopping mall to visit Santa. Some days later his teacher was telling me about the trip and commenting that he loved fries. She had given him fries from the McDonald's at the mall. My first reaction was horror at the fact that she had introduced my son to the very symbol of junk food! Then I thought, "Wait a minute, he ate them?" my son who only ate a handful of things, with a particular texture. Until he was three years old I had to purée his food. I think it was then that I allowed myself a faint glimmer of hope that this massage might actually help him. Those fries represented a major step in a long journey for us.

At the end of the five months, he was wearing socks, tantrums were less frequent both at home and at school, he was sleeping much better and had even started playing around with words to make simple jokes! Two years later, we still do qigong massage several times a week. It seems to help him.

I would tell new parents, QST works! It has been tested in many studies. There's not much you can do wrong with it, all you have to do is spend a few minutes every day with your child, and that time together is very special.

Many thanks,

Sarah

Weekly Log - Week 25

♥ Always start with love

Check each day you do the massage

Sun ___ Mon ___ Tuesday ___ Wed ___ Thu ___ Fri ___ Sat ___

Things You Noticed:

During the Massage

Mv1. Lays down/won't lay down?

Mv2. Back – hums?

Mv3-4. Ears – avoids?

Mv5. Up/up/up – eye contact?

Mv6. Fingers – stroking or pressing?

Mv7. Chest – rubs eyes, yawns, relaxes?

Mv8. Belly – diarrhea/constipation?

Mv9-10. Legs – patting or pressing?

Mv11. Toes – stroking, pressing, bicycle?

Mv12. Soles – avoids?

During the Week

Sleep _____

Bowels _____

Tantrums _____

Affection _____

Eye contact _____

Listening _____

Speaking _____

Other_____

Positive things other people said about your child ...

Your thoughts and feelings about the process ...

Questions you had this week ...

Remember: Look for answers to your questions in the index and the book.

Week 26
Letter to parents – Widening social circles (siblings, grandparents, friends)

Dear Parents,

By now you may be seeing that your child is beginning to connect with other people more. Over the years, we have noticed that a child who is in QST recovery widens her social circle in a predictable way.

The center of the social circle is the parent-child relationship, and it starts at birth. One dad said: "When my daughter was born, she looked in my eyes and saw my soul. She has owned me ever since." This is the essential human connection - life affirming and life-sustaining.

If your child has started out closer to one parent, the next thing that will happen with QST parent massage is she will open up to the other parent. After that, she will open up to older siblings, and then younger siblings.

A mom had this to say about her young son and his baby sister:

> *"My son never really noticed his baby sister. He would even crawl right over her like she wasn't even there. Then I noticed that he started watching her play, and now he sits down next to her to play." - Father*

Next, children will open up to grandparents and extended family members with whom they are familiar. Lastly, they will open up to relationships with children their own age. Now they are ready for school. Congratulations, it's been a long haul!

Best wishes,

Louisa and Pam

Weekly Log - Week 26

♥ Always start with love

Check each day you do the massage

Sun ___ Mon ___ Tuesday ___ Wed ___ Thu ___ Fri ___ Sat ___

Things You Noticed:

During the Massage

Mv1. Lays down/won't lay down?

Mv2. Back – hums?

Mv3-4. Ears – avoids?

Mv5. Up/up/up – eye contact?

Mv6. Fingers – stroking or pressing?

Mv7. Chest – rubs eyes, yawns, relaxes?

Mv8. Belly – diarrhea/constipation?

Mv9-10. Legs – patting or pressing?

Mv11. Toes – stroking, pressing, bicycle?

Mv12. Soles – avoids?

During the Week

Sleep _____

Bowels _____

Tantrums _____

Affection _____

Eye contact _____

Listening _____

Speaking _____

Other_____

Positive things other people said about your child ...

Your thoughts and feelings about the process ...

Questions you had this week ...

Remember: Look for answers to your questions in the index and the book.

Week 27

Letter to parents – How do I talk to the school about QST massage?

Dear Parents,

Chances are your child's teacher will be asking you what you are doing at home long before you go to talk to them! We often find that within a short time of starting QST massage, parents receive positive reports from the school. And teachers want to know what is happening. After all, they have a whole classroom full of children to teach, and something that helps one child, can help others too.

When your child's teacher asks you what you are doing, go ahead and give them the Information Sheet for teachers in Appendix 1. They will want to know about the research and what it showed.

We do not recommend that you teach the massage to your child's teacher or give them permission to give your child massage in school. You have spent a lot of time developing your child's trust in the massage. If school personnel are not sensitive to your child's body language or force the massage on your child, it can undermine your hard won goals. You can, however, share the transitions technique with your child's teacher and even show them how to use the Easy Button to calm your child and the Face-Me Button to get their attention. Teachers will be very glad to have these tools to support your child.

Keep up the good work!

Louisa and Pam

Weekly Log - Week 27

♥ Always start with love

Check each day you do the massage

Sun ___ Mon ___ Tuesday ___ Wed ___ Thu ___ Fri ___ Sat ___

Things You Noticed:

During the Massage

Mv1. Lays down/won't lay down?

Mv2. Back – hums?

Mv3-4. Ears – avoids?

Mv5. Up/up/up – eye contact?

Mv6. Fingers – stroking or pressing?

Mv7. Chest – rubs eyes, yawns, relaxes?

Mv8. Belly – diarrhea/constipation?

Mv9-10. Legs – patting or pressing?

Mv11. Toes – stroking, pressing, bicycle?

Mv12. Soles – avoids?

During the Week

Sleep _____

Bowels _____

Tantrums _____

Affection _____

Eye contact _____

Listening _____

Speaking _____

Other_____

Positive things other people said about your child ...

Your thoughts and feelings about the process ...

Questions you had this week ...

Remember: Look for answers to your questions in the index and the book.

Week 28

Letter to parents – How do I talk to my doctor about QST Massage?

Dear Parents,

Doctors are very open to treatments that can safely be given at home to young children with disabilities, and they are well aware that parent touch is important for the developing child.

Our experience telling doctors about QST massage for autism is that they see it as a win-win. It is natural, it doesn't have side effects, and it involves touch - something that doctors know children need, and parents do anyway.

They won't be surprised to learn that your child sleeps better with massage, is more relaxed and has less tantrums. It will make sense with what they already know to be true about the importance of touch. They will be surprised to learn that your child is more social and more receptive to communication. QST massage is new, and most doctors are not yet aware of the research showing that it is an effective treatment for autism.

Doctors are open to learning about treatments that are supported by research. Take your doctor the Information Sheet for your child's doctor in Appendix 2 and share what QST massage has done for your child. Your doctor will be curious about your experience and interested in the research. He or she will think about it, and possibly pass the information on to other families in need. Because of you, other children may receive help from the massage, too.

All the best,

Louisa and Pam

Weekly Log - Week 28

♥ Always start with love

Check each day you do the massage

Sun ___ Mon ___ Tuesday ___ Wed ___ Thu ___ Fri ___ Sat ___

Things You Noticed:

During the Massage

Mv1. Lays down/won't lay down?

Mv2. Back – hums?

Mv3-4. Ears – avoids?

Mv5. Up/up/up – eye contact?

Mv6. Fingers – stroking or pressing?

Mv7. Chest – rubs eyes, yawns, relaxes?

Mv8. Belly – diarrhea/constipation?

Mv9-10. Legs – patting or pressing?

Mv11. Toes – stroking, pressing, bicycle?

Mv12. Soles – avoids?

During the Week

Sleep _____

Bowels _____

Tantrums _____

Affection _____

Eye contact _____

Listening _____

Speaking _____

Other_____

Positive things other people said about your child ...

Your thoughts and feelings about the process ...

Questions you had this week ...

Remember: Look for answers to your questions in the index and the book.

Week 29
Letter to parents – A mother's feelings

Dear parents and caregivers,

You are amazing. Your work with your child is amazing. How can I know this without knowing you? Because after sixteen years of parenting a child with severe autism, I know that your daily reality is so full of highs and lows, small victories and enduring challenges, that the only way you can stay alive is with an open heart. We are all haunted by the idea that we aren't doing enough for our child. But you are doing something with this massage, and hundreds of other things each day, that are very good for your child and for you.

Our son, Jordon, was one of the first to receive this massage. He was the pilot light for the pilot study of Qigong massage more than fourteen years ago. A lot of water has passed under the bridge since then. He has had many ups and downs, most of which I could not have predicted when he first started the massage. The massage helped him open to others. It helped him communicate. It helped him be more grounded in his body. But it didn't "fix" everything. Because the challenges will continue both during the massage and after, I wanted to write this letter to you, to encourage you. I wanted you to know some of the reasons I think it is all worth it.

The other night when I went in to say goodnight to Jordan, I paused by the side of his bed. All of the sudden I was seized with a realization of just how much he has to put up with in any given day just to navigate his way through the world. Every day people misunderstand him, including me. Every day he has to be patient with not being able to fully communicate his needs and desires or his thoughts or dreams, even with me. Every day he has to watch as other people react negatively to him, sometimes with frustration, including me.

I am struck by his quiet dignity. He is so happy most of the time, and yet he does not "get" most of the things the world says make us happy. I know I often approach him with my own agendas - to teach him, guide him, direct him, fix him. Sometimes amidst all the therapies and programs we have for autism, amidst the stress of life with autism, we sometimes forget to simply sit back in awe and appreciate the beauty and dignity of the person who is our child. Sitting with that awe and appreciation allows me to be able to continue to give.

There are things about Jordan at sixteen that I love that I had no inkling of when he was three and starting massage. He has the best laugh ever - it lights up a room, it's honest and free. As one of our friends says, "There is nothing better than Jordan happy." I like to think of his laugh as a window into his soul. All children have these windows, the little places where you can see the expansive nature of their souls. As a parent, I need to pause when I hear Jordan's laugh and think, "What a large and generous soul." I need to be reminded of this so my gaze isn't just on his limits, or mine.

I had no idea that Jordan's hardest times were the times that would bring us closer together as a family. Two years ago, he was so aggressive we had to send him to foster care for a summer. It was one of the hardest things our family has ever done. After we had healed and after he had learned, we were ready to bring him home and we have grown closer. Our family is stronger than I could have ever known if there had never been a Jordan.

I love taking him out now - on walks, to the store, downtown. When he was younger it was a challenge. But now we go everywhere together. He loves it. What I love the most is watching other people react to him. It is absolutely astonishing to me how kind many people are. Yes, there are unkind people, too, but Jordan's generosity of spirit allows me to feel compassion for them instead of anger.

Jordan helps us to be free. I say this even knowing that having a child with autism means that there are many, many limits to what we can do, and to what he can do. These limits are sometimes unbelievably frustrating. But he helps us to see that sometimes our greatest freedom is found by living within our limits. Our notions of success or what is important do not matter to him. What he cares most about is that we love him and each other. Loving Jordan has let us see that nothing - no person, no disability, no strange noise or movement, no odd or aggressive behavior, no lack of skill or success, no challenge - is outside of love.

Sincerely, Lori

Weekly Log - Week 29

♥ Always start with love

Check each day you do the massage

Sun ___ Mon ___ Tuesday ___ Wed ___ Thu ___ Fri ___ Sat ___

Things You Noticed:

During the Massage

Mv1. Lays down/won't lay down?

Mv2. Back – hums?

Mv3-4. Ears – avoids?

Mv5. Up/up/up – eye contact?

Mv6. Fingers – stroking or pressing?

Mv7. Chest – rubs eyes, yawns, relaxes?

Mv8. Belly – diarrhea/constipation?

Mv9-10. Legs – patting or pressing?

Mv11. Toes – stroking, pressing, bicycle?

Mv12. Soles – avoids?

During the Week

Sleep _____

Bowels _____

Tantrums _____

Affection _____

Eye contact _____

Listening _____

Speaking _____

Other_____

Positive things other people said about your child ...

Your thoughts and feelings about the process ...

Questions you had this week ...

Remember: Look for answers to your questions in the index and the book.

Week 30
Letter to parents – A father's feelings

Dear fathers,

You are the father of a child with autism. This is something you did not sign up for, but something that will define the rest of your life. Being a father will be among the most challenging, life-changing and potentially fulfilling aspects of your life. It will be hard, very hard – I'm not going to lie. You can also throw out the playbook that was in your head prior to becoming a parent of an autistic child. It is irrelevant now. Grieve for this loss, and you should, but then move forward.

There exists instead a relentlessness that will define many of the experiences that you will have with your son or daughter. The highs will be higher, and the lows will be lower – every day, every week, every year. My experiences fathering Michael, age 16, tell me that this will not change. That is okay. He is how he is supposed to be, and that is how I am to love him – with that same relentlessness that he himself demands out of life.

Why the massage? There is a power of touch that can only come from a father – a combination of strength, intimacy and understanding. Similar to the unique power of touch that emanates from the mother, many of the nuances of this power can only come from a father.

You have a great opportunity and responsibility to participate in the massage, a practice that can open up the possibilities of communication and relationship that, painfully, have probably not been evident to the extent of your hopes and dreams. Your strength, your love and your faith in your child can make you a key contributor to his wholeness.

Your reality as the parent of an autistic child is a stark invitation to live in the present – you will want to live in a past that no longer exists, and you will want to imagine a future that is not going to happen in any predictable way. The present is difficult; it is a 24/7 commitment. It is, though, full of life. And it is good.

The massage, along with an open heart, is an opportunity to draw closer to your child, to commit to embarking on an incredible, fulfilling, exhausting journey. It is a journey that will allow you to love ferociously, to appreciate the small and real things that make life meaningful, and to be an example of tolerance and acceptance to all those around you.

After 16 years, I am still confident that we come out the other side of our journey very much intact.

A father

Weekly Log - Week 30

♥ Always start with love

Check each day you do the massage

Sun ___ Mon ___ Tuesday ___ Wed ___ Thu ___ Fri ___ Sat ___

Things You Noticed:

During the Massage

Mv1. Lays down/won't lay down?

Mv2. Back – hums?

Mv3-4. Ears – avoids?

Mv5. Up/up/up – eye contact?

Mv6. Fingers – stroking or pressing?

Mv7. Chest – rubs eyes, yawns, relaxes?

Mv8. Belly – diarrhea/constipation?

Mv9-10. Legs – patting or pressing?

Mv11. Toes – stroking, pressing, bicycle?

Mv12. Soles – avoids?

During the Week

Sleep _____

Bowels _____

Tantrums _____

Affection _____

Eye contact _____

Listening _____

Speaking _____

Other_____

Positive things other people said about your child ...

Your thoughts and feelings about the process ...

Questions you had this week ...

Remember: Look for answers to your questions in the index and the book.

Week 31
Letter to parents – Parents talk about QST

Dear Parents,

This will be a little different kind of parent letter than the ones you're used to seeing. So far this year you've learned an awful lot about QST and your child. You've developed and perfected some new skills to help your child. You've assessed their progress through the first half year and re-set your goals for the next half year.

Then the last two weeks you heard one mother and one father share their feelings about their own journey through autism and QST. Over the coming weeks you'll hear stories from other families about their experiences. So, this week we thought we'd share comments we've heard from lots of different parents about how they've experienced the changes they've seen in their child with QST – and how their relationship with their child has changed as a result. s

- *"She is a lot more cuddly!"*
- *"Meltdowns are fewer and less severe. And he's using his words much more."*
- *"He has started to self-soothe. He tries new things, and is interested in more things than just matchbox cars!"*
- *"He is more cuddly and affectionate than before. He hugs and kisses his stuffed animals now, as well as gives his Dad and I more hugs and kisses."*
- *"He has grown up so much. It's amazing to see the transformation. The frustrated little boy who couldn't get his point across has finally come out, and he has so much to say and do!"*
- *"He can feel pain now. And he has stopped biting me!"*
- *"We've become closer, and he's developed a stronger bond with both his parents."*
- *"He is able to sleep during the night, his language has catapulted, and he is less aggressive."*

- *"Massage gets you and your kid closer. It's time to relax and show love to each other."*

- *"We saw changes right away. His language increased as well as his awareness of what was happening in his environment. He began to understand much more and communicate more effectively. His frustrations and tantrums decreased as his communication and understanding increased. He seems more motivated to communicate. And his focus has greatly improved."*

- *"It's brought us closer. We both really enjoy the time we spend doing the massage together. It's been a real bonding experience for us. It's also a good time for both of us to de-stress and calm down together."*

- *"He has always cuddled with his Dad, but has been very selective cuddling with me. Now he approaches me, wants me, asks for me, and it feels like he loves me whereas before it did not."*

- *"Before the massage when his Dad and I hugged, kissed and snuggled him, he responded by "allowing" us to "assault" him – at least that's how it felt. He would stare off away from us. Now he is reciprocating, and will even seeks hugs and comfort. That is the most significant change for us!"*

- *"All around vast improvements in every area I can think of!"*

Now we'll close with a few quotes from parents as they sum up their experience of QST as a whole.

- *"It's done by me and my husband. No outsider can do it better than we can. Every other improvement seems to be because of some professional. This is because of our touch."*

- *"Overall, he is so much happier, calmer, and life is so much more enjoyable and livable."*

- *"This is something I can do at home any time, and it's easy to do. I can also tailor it to his individual issues. It really does make a difference, and it's so worth the time you put into it!"*

- *"Qigong is the only treatment he's had that has shown a significant difference in his behavior."*

- *"I think Qigong has complimented the speech and occupational therapy services he's had."*
- *"I love that the massage focused on strengthening his skills and working on him being comfortable in his own body."*
- *"This is about touch and energy and doing something for him, not asking him to do something for us, like speech therapy."*
- *"It's fun!"*
- *"I feel more empowered."*
- *"The massage is parent delivered. All the other methods for his autism are done by others. It is intimate and I feel like I am taking an active part."*
- *"It's gentle, safe and fosters our relationship with him."*
- *"It is easy and something I can do at home. It's been what's made all the other therapies work. It has done more for him than speech and OT. It was like they didn't work until we started the massage."*
- *"It is something I can do for him and see the changes daily."*
- *"The massage is every day, like a medicine. It's easy to put into a routine. It has been a positive experience from start to finish and has given us nothing but rewards."*
- *"It's family-oriented, it's long-term, it's inexpensive, it has no risks. It makes you feel that you have some control in an uncontrollable situation."*

We hope you've enjoyed hearing from so many different parents and feel some of the excitement and hope we do when we read these remarks. Now take out your Weekly Log and add your own comments about your own experience. Have fun!

Louisa and Pam

Weekly Log - Week 31

♥ Always start with love

Check each day you do the massage

Sun ___ Mon ___ Tuesday ___ Wed ___ Thu ___ Fri ___ Sat ___

Things You Noticed:

During the Massage

Mv1. Lays down/won't lay down?

Mv2. Back – hums?

Mv3-4. Ears – avoids?

Mv5. Up/up/up – eye contact?

Mv6. Fingers – stroking or pressing?

Mv7. Chest – rubs eyes, yawns, relaxes?

Mv8. Belly – diarrhea/constipation?

Mv9-10. Legs – patting or pressing?

Mv11. Toes – stroking, pressing, bicycle?

Mv12. Soles – avoids?

During the Week

Sleep _____

Bowels _____

Tantrums _____

Affection _____

Eye contact _____

Listening _____

Speaking _____

Other_____

Positive things other people said about your child ...

Your thoughts and feelings about the process ...

Questions you had this week ...

Remember: Look for answers to your questions in the index and the book.

Week 32

Letter to parents – Jilia's story – QST massage helped us through emotionally hard times

Dear Parents,

I'm so grateful for Qigong and to have this chance to share with other parents just how much it has helped my daughter and me through some really hard times in our family.

To make a long story short, my husband and I divorced when Jilia was just a year old. Unfortunately, it was one of those horrible, devastating divorces that involved a really vicious custody battle that lasted for years.

My precious daughter, who was already struggling with symptoms of autism, bore the brunt of the conflict, a long drawn-out custody battle and relentless manipulation by the very adults who were supposed to be her source of security and comfort. She even ended up being diagnosed with PTSD as a result. My heart just breaks when I consider what we went through during those years. We were both pretty broken.

A friend told me about Qigong massage, and told me Jilia and I really needed it! I believed her. She gave me the book and DVD, and I learned the massage and started doing it every single day except when Jilia was at her father's.

At first, her body was pretty rigid through most of the movements, especially in her neck and shoulders. Her fingers and toes were super sensitive. Her toes were so painful I could hardly touch them. But after only a few days, she was much more receptive to the whole massage. Her entire body seemed more relaxed.

I remember one day early on, Julia wanted to watch the DVD of Dr. Silva giving the massage, the one that comes with the book. I thought for sure she'd lose interest after 5 minutes, but she was entranced for the full 30 minutes! I think she especially liked watching the kids on the video getting the massage.

One thing that really bothered me is that Jilia would cry and become very emotional, especially with the feet at first, and then later with the chest and belly.

I mean, it was really heart-wrenching crying, and it was hard to watch and not to stop, I have to admit. I would sometimes cry myself, but I kept on doing the massage and telling her "You're okay, Jilia, you're okay," like the book says to do. It was hard. There was so much going on for her emotionally, but the massage helped her release a lot of grief and pain that she hadn't felt safe to release any other way. And she kept asking for it every day, so she knew on some level that it was helping her.

There was also a time when she had "night terrors," and would wake up in a panic screaming, "Momma! Where are you? Don't leave me!" over and over again. It was very disturbing. One night I felt an instinct to do Qigong massage with her in that moment. Her response was instant and she calmed right down, took huge deep breaths and fell fast asleep!

And of course there was a lot going on for me emotionally, too, during this time. Sometimes I felt so much shame that she wasn't with me more and I was always an emotional mess when she had to leave to go to her Dad's.

But within a few months, Jilia was so much more relaxed, and her whole body would just "let go" the minute we started the massage. She would unconsciously sigh, and as the giver of the Qigong I felt much more confident and able to feel her energy and responses and offer her love, feeling and healthy energy. There is a very special bonding that happens that is very intimate between us. Jilia says she likes being touched by her Momma, that it makes her feel good and calm. We're both healing.

One huge physical difference was in her swimming. It was as if something finally connected her body and mind. One day I was moved to tears watching her glide across the pool in freestyle. She had never swam that well, so in sync with stroke, body placement in the water, breathing, strength. She was beautiful!

Another time she had to have two teeth extracted and nearly flipped out in the dentist chair. I quietly did qigong on her lower limbs as she lay in the chair and whispered to her that I was helping her to ground in our "special" way with love and breath. She knew what I was doing, and she settled down while the dentist worked on her.

A year into Qigong massage, Julia had overcome a lot of her anxiety and fears and was having so many successes on so many levels in school, in sports, and in her own feelings and emotions. Three years into it, I was overcome with gratitude and joy that she has come through a long emotionally exhausting time and is happy, confident and independent. We're now five years in, and yes, we still do Qigong. We both love it and it helps both of us feel calm and centered.

Qigong is and has been amazing for Jilia and totally supported her recovery from trauma and PTSD, and helped her learn many tools she still incorporates today as coping skills when the world and its energies drain her completely. We both learned so much, I am so grateful that I learned to give Julia Qigong, and I hope other parents love this as much as we do.

Yours truly,

Jilia's Mom

Weekly Log - Week 32

♥ Always start with love

Check each day you do the massage

Sun ___ Mon ___ Tuesday ___ Wed ___ Thu ___ Fri ___ Sat ___

Things You Noticed:

During the Massage

Mv1. Lays down/won't lay down?

Mv2. Back – hums?

Mv3-4. Ears – avoids?

Mv5. Up/up/up – eye contact?

Mv6. Fingers – stroking or pressing?

Mv7. Chest – rubs eyes, yawns, relaxes?

Mv8. Belly – diarrhea/constipation?

Mv9-10. Legs – patting or pressing?

Mv11. Toes – stroking, pressing, bicycle?

Mv12. Soles – avoids?

During the Week

Sleep _____

Bowels _____

Tantrums _____

Affection _____

Eye contact _____

Listening _____

Speaking _____

Other_____

Positive things other people said about your child ...

Your thoughts and feelings about the process ...

Questions you had this week ...

Remember: Look for answers to your questions in the index and the book.

Week 33
Reflections from a Master Trainer

Dear Parents,

Welcome to QST. You are beginning this journey with our medicine because you have already been baptized by fire – your child is in need of all the support you can summon, and you are keenly aware how much your child's future depends on you. Simply knowing that it is in your hands to make the best, most heartfelt decisions about what is right and good for your child is not the same thing as having a tool in your hands to help you advance down that path. With QST, we give you a tool in your hands – hands that are always with you and already know how to help your child.

Welcome to relief! While the first days may be trying and even exasperating, soon you will see the change coming. You will know that your daily devotion to your child makes a difference. Maybe the change will be simple – sounder sleep or less crankiness. Maybe it will be profound – first words or a true gaze into your eyes, signaling connection. However it unfolds for your family, trust that there are enough families who have been down this path already and who can attest to the power of their experience with QST.

As a Master Trainer, I am here to help you. I am a Master not because I am especially capable, but because I can hold for you the belief that this will help you and your child, even while you may still be wondering whether it will. I believe that you are gifted – in the midst of your worry and probably exhaustion, you are replete with commitment. That commitment is the medicine that you will transfer through your hands to the body of your child, and it will nourish your entire family in the process.

We are so fortunate to do this work, to engage with parents like you. I hope you will approach the glimmer of optimism you may feel in reading our letters as an invitation to hope – because we stand for that on your behalf.

Warmly,

A QST Master Trainer

Weekly Log - Week 33

♥ Always start with love

Check each day you do the massage

Sun ___ Mon ___ Tuesday ___ Wed ___ Thu ___ Fri ___ Sat ___

Things You Noticed:

During the Massage

Mv1. Lays down/won't lay down?

Mv2. Back – hums?

Mv3-4. Ears – avoids?

Mv5. Up/up/up – eye contact?

Mv6. Fingers – stroking or pressing?

Mv7. Chest – rubs eyes, yawns, relaxes?

Mv8. Belly – diarrhea/constipation?

Mv9-10. Legs – patting or pressing?

Mv11. Toes – stroking, pressing, bicycle?

Mv12. Soles – avoids?

During the Week

Sleep _____

Bowels _____

Tantrums _____

Affection _____

Eye contact _____

Listening _____

Speaking _____

Other_____

Positive things other people said about your child ...

Your thoughts and feelings about the process ...

Questions you had this week ...

Remember: Look for answers to your questions in the index and the book.

Week 34

Letter to parents – Reflections from a Chinese Grandmother

Dear Parents,

I was a retired math teacher living in Shangai, China before I moved to the U.S. My older son, who has worked with Dr. Silva for many years, introduced me to her ten years ago when I first arrived in the U.S.

I have always been impressed by Dr. Silva's non-medicine therapy for children with autism. She based this treatment on the theory of Chinese medicine, and she involved parents in the daily treatment of their children. This therapy creates a strong emotional and physical connection between parents and their child, which is so important to families who have felt helpless in the face of the difficulties their children with autism face.

Dr. Silva has published many studies, using Western scientific research standards, including a multi-year study funded by a federal research grant. I admire and respect Dr. Silva's hard work, attitude and confidence in Chinese medicine as a doctor of Western medicine. She draws from both traditions. She uses knowledge of Chinese medicine in creating and understanding how this therapy works, and uses knowledge from western medicine in testing its effectiveness and improving it.

Dr. Silva has put her love, responsibility and life's work into this method. She has made a beautiful contribution to the promotion and expansion of Chinese medicine in western countries. She is also extending her method to other countries to help more families and children.

I feel sad that there is no doctor studying this traditional method in China now. China has the biggest population in the world, and there are more and more children being diagnosed with autism there now. Dr. Silva has translated her book and materials into Chinese and will be offering parent and therapist training in China. Chinese families who have children with autism need help, and I am heartened that more Chinese families can find hope and benefit from this important therapy in the same ways that western families have.

A Chinese Grandmother

Weekly Log - Week 34

♥ Always start with love

Check each day you do the massage

Sun ___ Mon ___ Tuesday ___ Wed ___ Thu ___ Fri ___ Sat ___

Things You Noticed:

During the Massage

Mv1. Lays down/won't lay down?

Mv2. Back – hums?

Mv3-4. Ears – avoids?

Mv5. Up/up/up – eye contact?

Mv6. Fingers – stroking or pressing?

Mv7. Chest – rubs eyes, yawns, relaxes?

Mv8. Belly – diarrhea/constipation?

Mv9-10. Legs – patting or pressing?

Mv11. Toes – stroking, pressing, bicycle?

Mv12. Soles – avoids?

During the Week

Sleep _____

Bowels _____

Tantrums _____

Affection _____

Eye contact _____

Listening _____

Speaking _____

Other_____

Positive things other people said about your child ...

Your thoughts and feelings about the process ...

Questions you had this week ...

Remember: Look for answers to your questions in the index and the book.

Week 35

Letter to parents – William's story – recovery from autism

Dear Parents,

My son William came into the world brilliant and braced against connection. He was sensitive from his earliest days. Unlike other children whose autism came over them like a wave after they'd already learned to stand on their own, William was in retreat from the moment he arrived. He loved us fiercely but wouldn't let us hold him. He felt deeply but rarely spoke. He was a strong presence but not a participant.

When William was 3 years old, he attempted pre-school. We enrolled him in an integrated program that combined children on the spectrum with typically developing children. I anticipated that this would lead to a proper assessment and meaningful support. Unfortunately, William's anxiety overshadowed his autism and the program only reinforced his fearfulness of the new, strange and overwhelming.

By the time he was 8, William was living in the "in-between" – not properly diagnosed, not receiving appropriate support, and miserable in his own skin. That's when I learned about QST. From the first massage he started to come into himself in a way that was new to all of us. He immediately became more talkative. His ability and willingness to be at ease with textures and sounds and stimulation that previously undid him came quickly. We made great progress, and we had a new hopefulness about his future.

About two months into the massage, William shifted again. He had a loss in his life that was hard to absorb. A person dear to him had moved away. William became depressed, and the massage made it possible, I believe, for him to feel his grief. For a time he came apart, like any child does when they experience such a loss, but the tidal wave of feelings that washed up with the grief had deeper, older origins in his life. I feared I had made an unforgiveable mistake in exposing him to his own raw emotions. It took strong coaching from our QST therapist to allow ourselves to push on with the only intervention that had really helped William so far.

Over time, and with additional support, William grew through the despair and grew up to be a fine teen who can feel his feelings and be with his family. No one who knew him then would recognize him now. He does not qualify for an autism diagnosis. He is open, funny, often silly, and still brilliant. We are grateful for what QST did for him and our family.

William's Mom

Weekly Log - Week 35

♥ Always start with love

Check each day you do the massage

Sun ___ Mon ___ Tuesday ___ Wed ___ Thu ___ Fri ___ Sat ___

Things You Noticed:

During the Massage

Mv1. Lays down/won't lay down?

Mv2. Back – hums?

Mv3-4. Ears – avoids?

Mv5. Up/up/up – eye contact?

Mv6. Fingers – stroking or pressing?

Mv7. Chest – rubs eyes, yawns, relaxes?

Mv8. Belly – diarrhea/constipation?

Mv9-10. Legs – patting or pressing?

Mv11. Toes – stroking, pressing, bicycle?

Mv12. Soles – avoids?

During the Week

Sleep _____

Bowels _____

Tantrums _____

Affection _____

Eye contact _____

Listening _____

Speaking _____

Other_____

Positive things other people said about your child ...

Your thoughts and feelings about the process ...

Questions you had this week ...

Remember: Look for answers to your questions in the index and the book.

Week 36
Letter to parents – Cognitive impairment – the thing we can't change

Dear Parents,

Much of autism research focuses on the brain as the cause of developmental delay. We think that developmental delay occurs because the brain does not get normal information from the senses. In most children, once the sensory problems are taken care of, development starts catching up. We also think that in a smaller percentage of children, whatever caused the sensory problems may also have harmed the brain. One of the questions parents are often afraid to ask is, "Will my child end up with cognitive (mental) impairment?"

It is impossible to know which children will end up with cognitive impairment. Just because a pre-school child is severely autistic at age 3, doesn't mean they will stay severely autistic – they might end up with moderate, or mild autism, or maybe they will eventually grow out of it. Severity of autism is usually classified according to how severe the behavior is and how delayed the language. We are not as worried about severe behavior - we have found that behavior problems are mostly due to sensory issues and can resolve quite well with massage. But we do think the most worrisome sign of severity is lack of language that persists after a year or two of massage.

We have worked with many 3-5 year olds who had little or no speech when they started qigong massage. Testing usually shows they are in the bottom 30% of language skills for their age. But for most of them, speech improves with qigong massage - by the end of the first year, they might be at 50% of expected language skills for their age, and by the end of the second year, they might be at 65%. Their language makes progress with massage. But there are some children whose language never really progresses with massage. Other things improve - sensory problems, behavior and parenting stress - but language does not come in. In our view these are the children who may have cognitive impairment.

We cannot know starting out which children will have cognitive impairment. But we do know how parents of children who did not develop language felt at the end of two years of massage. Even though they were disappointed that their child had not developed language, they felt it had been worth the time and energy they put into it. The behavioral and sensory problems had improved, it had brought them closer to their child, and it had made parenting easier.

> *"Our son hasn't started to talk yet, and we're not sure when he will. But we have a better understanding of our son now, and we are a lot less stressed about him." - Dad*

In the end, we don't know how things will end up. But we can always do our best with what we know, and that is what you are doing. We applaud you for it.

Respectfully,

Louisa and Pam

Weekly Log - Week 36

♥ Always start with love

Check each day you do the massage

Sun ___ Mon ___ Tuesday ___ Wed ___ Thu ___ Fri ___ Sat ___

Things You Noticed:

During the Massage

Mv1. Lays down/won't lay down?

Mv2. Back – hums?

Mv3-4. Ears – avoids?

Mv5. Up/up/up – eye contact?

Mv6. Fingers – stroking or pressing?

Mv7. Chest – rubs eyes, yawns, relaxes?

Mv8. Belly – diarrhea/constipation?

Mv9-10. Legs – patting or pressing?

Mv11. Toes – stroking, pressing, bicycle?

Mv12. Soles – avoids?

During the Week

Sleep _____

Bowels _____

Tantrums _____

Affection _____

Eye contact _____

Listening _____

Speaking _____

Other_____

Positive things other people said about your child ...

Your thoughts and feelings about the process ...

Questions you had this week ...

Remember: Look for answers to your questions in the index and the book.

Week 37

Letter to parents – Tom's story – a child with severe autism

Dear parents,

My son was very severe when we started the massage. He was four years old, he had no language, and he was wild. He didn't listen to us at all. He would get into a room and turn it upside down in a few minutes. He would run circles, looking up at the ceiling, not looking where he was going. We couldn't go anywhere with him. Someone had to be with him at all times.

We saw a lot of changes the first year we did the massage. He started making eye contact and listening to us. He calmed down a lot. We could tell him to put his shoes on, and he would go and get his shoes. In the mornings, while we were still in bed, he would peek around the bedroom door until we noticed him, and then scamper into bed with us. He is very close and affectionate now.

We didn't have as many changes the second year, and it was hard for me to accept that his growth was going to be so slow. I wanted him to start talking so badly! But I am more at peace with his progress now. I can see it happening bit by bit. He is a lot better. He doesn't tantrum anymore. We can take him to a restaurant and everyone can have a good time. He listens to us. We even went on a family vacation, and his behavior was fine.

I recommend this to all parents with children with autism. It made a huge difference to us.

Sincerely,

Tom's Dad

Weekly Log - Week 37

♥ Always start with love

Check each day you do the massage

Sun ___ Mon ___ Tuesday ___ Wed ___ Thu ___ Fri ___ Sat ___

Things You Noticed:

During the Massage

Mv1. Lays down/won't lay down?

Mv2. Back – hums?

Mv3-4. Ears – avoids?

Mv5. Up/up/up – eye contact?

Mv6. Fingers – stroking or pressing?

Mv7. Chest – rubs eyes, yawns, relaxes?

Mv8. Belly – diarrhea/constipation?

Mv9-10. Legs – patting or pressing?

Mv11. Toes – stroking, pressing, bicycle?

Mv12. Soles – avoids?

During the Week

Sleep _____

Bowels _____

Tantrums _____

Affection _____

Eye contact _____

Listening _____

Speaking _____

Other_____

Positive things other people said about your child ...

Your thoughts and feelings about the process ...

Questions you had this week ...

Remember: Look for answers to your questions in the index and the book.

Week 38

Letter to parents – Reflections from a Master Trainer: QST balances the neurotransmitters

Dear Parents,

I have worked as an OT for 45 years. I took Dr. Silva's training in QST massage ten years ago. I have seen many amazing things in the children we have treated.

I want to share with you what Dr. Silva says about QST, "It needs to be given every day, like a medicine." And I want to explain "Why."

Children's brains learn when they are relaxed and open. That is why we aim for relaxation during massage. Stress tends to shut brain learning down.

At night during sleep, the brain de-stresses, processes the day's learning and integrates the new into the old. It combines experiences together and finds the hidden rules. That is why you might wake up having solved a problem in your sleep.

Children with autism are easily stressed and fall into three brain and behavior patterns:

- Fear: the child holds still and doesn't respond to the world around him
- Fright: child screams at any attempt to move him from the situation he is in
- Flight: the child runs away from the situation because he feels threatened

The nerve pathways are present in autism but the neurotransmitters are not working properly. Neurotransmitters are substances that carry a signal from one nerve cell to another. A message might come from the outside world and head up towards the brain. Along the way the message has to be relayed from one nerve to another by neurotransmitters - like the wind carries a football from one player to the next. When the neurotransmitters are not working properly, our brains get a jumbled message.

Some of the major neurotransmitters that regulate behavior are:

- Serotonin: it is like the orchestra leader, it regulates the others
- Norepinephrine: it releases a sudden burst of energy in response to stress.

136

It can unbalance the other neurotransmitters

- Cortisol: is secreted with stress and can stop other messages from reaching the brain
- Dopamine: it is important for movement, happiness, motivation and memory
- GABA: it counterbalances excitation in the brain

For your child to have optimal brain function, the neurotransmitters must be balanced and orchestrated. A child with autism is not able to utilize neurotransmitters as a typical child does. The neurotransmitters are out of balance and information is difficult to process. That is why learning is delayed.

QST massage uses ancient Chinese massage techniques to send organized messages to the brain through the skin. This balances the neurotransmitters in your child's body and brain. This is why a daily dose of the massage is needed. When your child gets the massage, she can process the new learning in her sleep and wake up ready to learn more the next day.

Remember, your child is not only working on balancing his neurotransmitters, but growing, developing and picking up pieces of development that were missed - that is a lot of new learning for your child's brain! At some point your child's body will be able to adjust his own neurotransmitters on a daily basis and QST massage can be decreased. This process can take 2 to 3 years or 6 months. It is totally dependent on the child's needs.

But until your child can regulate himself on a daily basis, his brain will learn better if you give him the massage every day.

Sincerely,

Linda

Weekly Log - Week 38

♥ Always start with love

Check each day you do the massage

Sun ___ Mon ___ Tuesday ___ Wed ___ Thu ___ Fri ___ Sat ___

Things You Noticed:

During the Massage

Mv1. Lays down/won't lay down?

Mv2. Back – hums?

Mv3-4. Ears – avoids?

Mv5. Up/up/up – eye contact?

Mv6. Fingers – stroking or pressing?

Mv7. Chest – rubs eyes, yawns, relaxes?

Mv8. Belly – diarrhea/constipation?

Mv9-10. Legs – patting or pressing?

Mv11. Toes – stroking, pressing, bicycle?

Mv12. Soles – avoids?

During the Week

Sleep _____

Bowels _____

Tantrums _____

Affection _____

Eye contact _____

Listening _____

Speaking _____

Other_____

Positive things other people said about your child ...

Your thoughts and feelings about the process ...

Questions you had this week ...

Remember: Look for answers to your questions in the index and the book.

Week 39

Letter to parents – What QST massage has done for my son and my whole family

Dear Parents,

My son Josh is doing well in school now. When we started qigong, he was just beginning first grade. He was refusing to read. We knew he had a vocabulary and knew what the words meant, but as far as absorbing material from a book, he couldn't do it. By the end of first grade, we got him to pick up his first book. Now he is in second grade, and he is reading at 6th grade level and doing 3rd grade math.

Now he'd like to have his own youtube channel, and we're working on how to accomplish that! We have lots of stuff in store for him, and he has lots of stuff in store for himself. Now he tells us his dreams and goals, and what he wants to accomplish in life. I thought he was going to live with us for the rest of his life and be dependent on us. Now he is thinking about what kind of job he will have when he gets married. He is eight!

He has grown by leaps and bounds. He engages with people, makes eye contact, has full conversations, and allows certain individuals to pat him on the back. It has been real exciting because now he'll talk to people and not pull away. He'll look people in the eye. His school team is rejoicing.

Socially, he prefers adults much more than children. I think he considers himself a mini adult. If there were no other children at school, or a select few that he enjoys, it would be perfect. But he will approach other children now and try to engage them in play, which is monumental. But it is all on his terms. When kids get into his space, or push his bubble or are too noisy, he still has a challenge.

He is extremely close with me and with his siblings. This past year has been a difficult one for our family as we have gone through a very stressful custody battle. My son has been a trooper through this. He was aware of what was going on and understood what was happening.

139

He could sense when I was struggling and he would curl up next to me and snuggle. He did it with his little sister, too, and he wrestles and snuggles with his big brother now. He is also close to his grandpa. He doesn't like his grandpa touching him as much, but they will sit and play for hours and have in-depth conversations.

The massage has helped me understand when my children are distressed and has given me a way to bring them out of distress and back to being open. All my children have physical and behavioral challenges including sensory issues, autism and traumatic brain injury. But I wouldn't change any of my kids for the world. I am so much wiser now that I know we can work through distress, and I embrace their difficulties.

The qigong started the process of me learning about them and what they needed. And it's a foundational skill that I still use. Qigong has taught me about reading my children's body language and knowing what to do to help them. Every day before school, if I see Josh is tense, I give him a 'mini' massage. I pat the top of his head, pat down his back, and squeeze down his arms to get him ready for the day. I can see the tension shaking out of him. He goes from being tense to being ready for the day.

The massage works, it definitely, definitely works. I've recommended it to other people. I'm really glad we learned it.

My kids keep me going. Whether it is that close bond with them, or whether it is my passion to keep us together, my kids have always been my focus. We have overcome so much and qigong opened the door. It's helped us keep our super close bond as a family.

Sincerely,

Josh's mother

Weekly Log - Week 39

♥ Always start with love

Check each day you do the massage

Sun ___ Mon ___ Tuesday ___ Wed ___ Thu ___ Fri ___ Sat ___

Things You Noticed:

During the Massage

Mv1. Lays down/won't lay down?

Mv2. Back – hums?

Mv3-4. Ears – avoids?

Mv5. Up/up/up – eye contact?

Mv6. Fingers – stroking or pressing?

Mv7. Chest – rubs eyes, yawns, relaxes?

Mv8. Belly – diarrhea/constipation?

Mv9-10. Legs – patting or pressing?

Mv11. Toes – stroking, pressing, bicycle?

Mv12. Soles – avoids?

During the Week

Sleep _____

Bowels _____

Tantrums _____

Affection _____

Eye contact _____

Listening _____

Speaking _____

Other_____

Positive things other people said about your child ...

Your thoughts and feelings about the process ...

Questions you had this week ...

Remember: Look for answers to your questions in the index and the book.

Week 40
Letter to parents – QST and sensory kids

Dear Parents,

Over the years, we've been asked a lot about Sensory kids - children with sensory issues who don't have autism, but who do have sensory issues and problems regulating their behavior. You may know some yourself, and their parents may be asking you about QST and their children.

It is a strange statistic that today as many as 1 in 5 children in the U.S. have sensory issues. This is not the case in France, where research shows that children are about 25% as irritable, anxious or aggressive as children in the U.S. In France, the government supports mothers staying home with their children the whole first year of their lives. We think this has something to do with these differences.

Reassuring touch is a balm for the nervous system. It relaxes the nervous system and helps it process sensory input. Sensory over-sensitivity is a sign that a child is not receiving enough of that balm when they need it.

Many children in the U.S. spend as much as 40 hours a week in daycare. In many daycare facilities, safe conduct policies discourage staff from touching children more than is necessary for basic child care. These policies are designed to minimize the potential for sexual abuse. Unfortunately, they have been extended beyond their intended purpose with the result that adults feel restricted in their ability to physically comfort children in their care. If a child falls down and bruises her knee, staff can feel reluctant to hold her and soothe her until she stops crying. It seems strange, but staff is sometimes actually prohibited from picking children up to soothe them. Instead, they are trained to talk the child through the upset. This approach is not developmentally appropriate for a young child who needs reassuring touch to calm down or the nervous system doesn't learn to self-soothe. Without reassuring touch, the child may never process the upset, and be a little more fearful on the playground after that.

Is there a way to not throw out the baby with the bathwater, so to speak? Yes, we think there is. We definitely have to protect our children from abuse, and we also have to reassure and soothe them when they get upset. It is not one or the other; we need to do both. Attuned, reassuring parent or caregiver touch when the child needs it is as necessary to growth and development as food and water.

So, what can you tell your working friends whose children have sensory issues? Make them aware of the research. They can talk to the adults who care for their children. And when they get their children home at night, they can give them the QST Massage for Sensory kids! It's somewhat different than the one you give, but just like it does for your child, it will bring their child's nervous system to balance before bedtime, treat the sensory issues and cement the bond between child and parent.

That's what we call a win-win!

Best wishes,

Louisa and Pam

Weekly Log - Week 40

♥ Always start with love

Check each day you do the massage

Sun ___ Mon ___ Tuesday ___ Wed ___ Thu ___ Fri ___ Sat ___

Things You Noticed:

During the Massage

Mv1. Lays down/won't lay down?

Mv2. Back – hums?

Mv3-4. Ears – avoids?

Mv5. Up/up/up – eye contact?

Mv6. Fingers – stroking or pressing?

Mv7. Chest – rubs eyes, yawns, relaxes?

Mv8. Belly – diarrhea/constipation?

Mv9-10. Legs – patting or pressing?

Mv11. Toes – stroking, pressing, bicycle?

Mv12. Soles – avoids?

During the Week

Sleep _____

Bowels _____

Tantrums _____

Affection _____

Eye contact _____

Listening _____

Speaking _____

Other_____

Positive things other people said about your child ...

Your thoughts and feelings about the process ...

Questions you had this week ...

Remember: Look for answers to your questions in the index and the book.

Week 41

Letter to parents – Andrew's story – autism and Crohn's disease

Dear parents,

What do you most deeply want for your kids? For me it is that they are healthy and reaching their greatest potential. With autism that vision becomes much reduced. You go from dreaming of them taking the world head on to just praying you can get them functional enough to manage. I have spent countless hours trying to unlock the potential I could see stuck inside my son. Qigong massage unlocked his potential, allowed him to access his own brain and for the first time to understand himself and how to connect with others. This is more than just another time commitment for parents, it's a life-altering tool. I am so blessed to have found it.

Andrew was born normal. When he was six months old he started waking up screaming in the night and nothing seemed to comfort him. Our pediatrician told us it was night terrors and not to worry, most kids grow out of it.

There were other challenges as he grew – we suspected lactose intolerance and eliminated milk from his diet; he would panic if I was out of his sight for even a second; the only word he spoke by the age of three was "Mama." His tantrums were terrible and could last for hours. The "night terrors" never really stopped. As he got more language, he would complain that his head hurt and scream until he vomited or passed out. He had severe seasonal allergies and bad diarrhea, sometimes with bleeding. His naturopath diagnosed dairy allergy, so we took him off dairy again and also gluten, and this seemed to help for awhile.

When he started kindergarten and ate all the snacks, candy and cookies other kids were eating, his digestive problems got really bad again. His doctor finally diagnosed Crohn's disease. His intestines and colon were a mess, and the doctor couldn't believe he was as relatively healthy as he was – she attributed that to all the good, healthy home cooking I'd been doing for him.

I was shocked to learn that Crohn's disease is not curable, that it can only be

145

managed – often with lots of medicine and even surgery if the drugs fail to keep it in remission. I removed everything from his diet that seemed to bother him and prepared very gentle, nutritious foods for him. With this and his medication, his Crohn's was stable but still seemed to be slowly getting worse over time.

About this time a client of my husband connected me to an online support group for families with children with special needs, including autism. One mother posted about Dr. Silva and Qigong massage. It was so interesting. I just knew this would do something for Andrew. And it has.

Soon after we started the massage, Andrew threw up a whole bunch of phlegm. I was worried that I had done something wrong! But Dr. Silva reassured me that when children detox it either goes up and out or down and out. Right afterwards, his little bloated belly got flat. He did a little more purging about three months into the massage. Then he regressed, but we were prepared for that. Andrew was in the Terrible Twos! It was difficult, with three other children and a new baby to have a 7 year old acting like a toddler. The good news is that it only lasted a week, and we made it through.

After that Andrew started healing and gaining weight. His cheeks got rosy, he started learning new things, he has his first growth spurt in years. He's started approaching and talking with other people on his own. He started saying rhyming words for the first time and actually sang a song out loud! I was amazed at the transformation! He seems to have a new learning of who he is and where he fits in this big bright world. And recently his lab results have been encouraging. They aren't perfect, but they are good enough to leave things be and his doctors are really surprised that he is getting better, not worse.

One day about four months into the massage, Andrew was struggling to get a fitted sheet on his mattress. I'd shown him many times how to do it, and I couldn't stop and help him because I was busy getting the other kids to bed, so I left him to figure it out on his own. Normally this would have ended in an epic meltdown, but instead he was able to calm himself down and to actually tell me, "I don't feel special, important to you, because you won't help me." I was so touched. He had never been able to articulate how he felt like that before. I had to choke back tears

146

as I put the boys on hold and went to help him. He really didn't need much help at all, and he was beaming and I was so proud of him! He hugged me so hard I couldn't breathe!

His Crohn's is doing very well now. We keep him on a diet, and he isn't sick with it anymore. He is growing like a weed!

Overall, he is a much different boy than when we started this journey. I know if I keep up the massage he will develop new skills and work through whatever continues to challenge him. This is more than a 15-30 minute commitment, it's the opportunity to breathe life into your child, an opportunity you are not likely to find elsewhere. I hope you find the person waiting to be unlocked inside your child, too!

A Mom

Weekly Log - Week 41

♥ Always start with love

Check each day you do the massage

Sun ___ Mon ___ Tuesday ___ Wed ___ Thu ___ Fri ___ Sat ___

Things You Noticed:

During the Massage

Mv1. Lays down/won't lay down?

Mv2. Back – hums?

Mv3-4. Ears – avoids?

Mv5. Up/up/up – eye contact?

Mv6. Fingers – stroking or pressing?

Mv7. Chest – rubs eyes, yawns, relaxes?

Mv8. Belly – diarrhea/constipation?

Mv9-10. Legs – patting or pressing?

Mv11. Toes – stroking, pressing, bicycle?

Mv12. Soles – avoids?

During the Week

Sleep _____

Bowels _____

Tantrums _____

Affection _____

Eye contact _____

Listening _____

Speaking _____

Other_____

Positive things other people said about your child ...

Your thoughts and feelings about the process ...

Questions you had this week ...

Remember: Look for answers to your questions in the index and the book.

Week 42
Letter to parents – A technique to encourage back-and-forth conversation

Dear Parents,

Some children we have worked with have quite a bit of language and can talk a long time about one thing – like a cartoon character – but without listening or even noticing that there is no back-and-forth conversation. And if you try to join their conversation, or have a different conversation with them, they don't know how to do this.

Here is an interesting story. A QST trainer and a mom were working with such a boy. He was lying on his back holding an action figure and talking about Sponge Bob. Mom was working on his belly and legs, and the trainer was up by his head. The boy was talking on and on about Sponge Bob and didn't seem to be aware of the massage at all.

The trainer wanted to break through to him, but she knew she couldn't use words – that wouldn't work. She had to use touch. She had to somehow reach the part of his brain that would make him want to listen and communicate. She knew about the direct connection from the hands to the speech part of the brain from her experience of doing movement 6, massaging the fingers until the lips move. And she thought about how she could send a very strong stimulus to both the right and the left side of the brain. She would have to strongly stimulate both hands at the same time.

So she began to apply firm in-and-out pressure from both elbows down to both hands, ending by squeezing both hands –about 60 squeezes per minute. She continued doing it – going back to the elbows when she finished the hands. He was quite relaxed with it. After about two minutes she asked him a question, and he didn't answer. But after about five minutes of squeezing down the arms, it was as if there was a little earthquake in him, and he shook down out of his head into his body, and he was present with the massage, his mom and the trainer in the

149

room. And then there was back-and-forth communication about his hands and the massage.

For children who are just starting to talk, we often recommend that parents do extra finger massage. But what we learned from that little boy, is that when you are doing extra outside of his daily massage because you want to help your child to communicate, it's sometimes helpful to massage both arms down to the hands at the same time. Don't plan to do this unless you can do it for five minutes or so, and you are relaxed. It's good to do when you are sitting with your child – it will help conversational sharing.

Good luck,

Louisa and Pam

Weekly Log - Week 42

♥ Always start with love

Check each day you do the massage

Sun ___ Mon ___ Tuesday ___ Wed ___ Thu ___ Fri ___ Sat ___

Things You Noticed:

During the Massage

Mv1. Lays down/won't lay down?

Mv2. Back – hums?

Mv3-4. Ears – avoids?

Mv5. Up/up/up – eye contact?

Mv6. Fingers – stroking or pressing?

Mv7. Chest – rubs eyes, yawns, relaxes?

Mv8. Belly – diarrhea/constipation?

Mv9-10. Legs – patting or pressing?

Mv11. Toes – stroking, pressing, bicycle?

Mv12. Soles – avoids?

During the Week

Sleep _____

Bowels _____

Tantrums _____

Affection _____

Eye contact _____

Listening _____

Speaking _____

Other_____

Positive things other people said about your child ...

Your thoughts and feelings about the process ...

Questions you had this week ...

Remember: Look for answers to your questions in the index and the book.

Week 43

Letter to parents – Qigong massage for the home medicine cabinet

Dear parents,

Although my two sons don't have autism, I still found the qigong massage invaluable!

I first used a short version of qigong massage when my youngest was just 2 months old. He was having problems latching during breastfeeding, causing me a lot of pain and him a lot of frustration. It completely amazed me that doing some specific qigong massage movements could help with latching issues. But it did!

When my youngest was three years old, he started having massive tantrums that often lasted three hours. It was miserable for the whole family! I happened to be learning the massage for my work at that time, so I decided to try it on my son to see what would happen. After a few weeks, the frequency and length of his tantrums decreased dramatically. After a while, he very rarely had a tantrum. So we started slacking and not doing the massage, then the tantrums came back! Once we resumed the massage, the tantrums went away again. This happened several times. So I'm certain that the massage made the difference!

Because I saw how much it helped, I ended up giving the massage to both of my sons at bedtime for a few years. For my older son, the massage was useful in helping him slow down from the day and get ready to sleep. His brain works very fast and hard, so getting him to unwind was challenging at times. But with the massage, it settled him right down.

Several years later, my boys occasionally still request that I give them qigong massage at bedtime. I think they can feel when their bodies need it.

The qigong massage was so helpful, even for my typically developing kiddos!

Mom of now 9-year-old and 12-year-old sons

Weekly Log - Week 43

♥ Always start with love

Check each day you do the massage

Sun ___ Mon ___ Tuesday ___ Wed ___ Thu ___ Fri ___ Sat ___

Things You Noticed:

During the Massage

Mv1. Lays down/won't lay down?

Mv2. Back – hums?

Mv3-4. Ears – avoids?

Mv5. Up/up/up – eye contact?

Mv6. Fingers – stroking or pressing?

Mv7. Chest – rubs eyes, yawns, relaxes?

Mv8. Belly – diarrhea/constipation?

Mv9-10. Legs – patting or pressing?

Mv11. Toes – stroking, pressing, bicycle?

Mv12. Soles – avoids?

During the Week

Sleep _____

Bowels _____

Tantrums _____

Affection _____

Eye contact _____

Listening _____

Speaking _____

Other_____

Positive things other people said about your child ...

Your thoughts and feelings about the process ...

Questions you had this week ...

Remember: Look for answers to your questions in the index and the book.

Week 44

The Four Risk Periods for Dropping the Massage

Dear parents,

We really want you to have success with the massage, and we want your children to benefit as much as possible from your hard work. Experience has taught us that there are four risk periods when parents who discontinue the massage are most likely to do so. Three out of the four have to do with the child changing or the parent needing to change the massage; one has to do with the child having less dramatic progress! We want you to be forewarned.

These are the four times:

Right at the beginning

If children have a lot of resistance when parents first start the program, parents can decide their child doesn't like the massage, or the massage doesn't work for their child.

Both of these are mistaken conclusions. If the child is struggling with the massage at the beginning, the parent hasn't yet found the right technique – the right speed and weight of their hand that can treat the child without triggering struggle. Here is what to do:

Decide you need to modify the massage technique. Review the book/DVD for suggestions, set up a distraction, and do the massage while they are watching a video. You can read more about this in Week 2.

After a few months

When children's sensory systems switch from under-sensitive to over-sensitive, they start feeling a lot more, their behavior can become challenging, and parents can decide that the massage has "stopped working," or is making their child worse.

Both of these would also be the wrong conclusions. When children switch from under-sensitive to over-sensitive, it is a huge sign of progress! You have been working towards this for some weeks. And guess what? The next stage after this one is normally sensitive – your goal. The over-sensitive stage lasts a few weeks, and if you modify the massage right away as soon as you notice it, you will help your child get through it faster and easier. A big tip-off that your child is entering this next stage is when they cry when they are injured for the first time. Read more about this in Weeks 3 and 21.

After a few more months

When the child suddenly moves into the Terrible Twos and for no apparent reason starts testing the parent and saying "no" a lot, sometimes parents can decide the massage has "stopped working" because the child's behavior is more challenging.

Again, this is the wrong conclusion. The truth is that the massage has now worked on the child's sensory system to the point that the child has come into an independent sense of self. The skin and the sense of touch are giving him information about his whole body, he can understand that he has a whole self, and now he can feel his will – and he wants to test it against yours! It's a very normal developmental stage and a wonderful achievement on your part! You just need to switch your parenting style now, and help him understand he has choices, but he doesn't control the world! See more tips about parenting this stage in Weeks 18 and 19.

At different times during the year

Other times the child's development smoothes out, and progress is no longer as dramatic as it was at the beginning. The child has come to relax and enjoy the massage, and massage can fall off the priority list because the parent decides that the child has benefited as much as they are going to from the massage.

You can probably guess by now that this, too, is the wrong conclusion! First of all, normal growth and development isn't particularly dramatic, and it often isn't the parent who lives with the child every day who notices the changes, but the relative who sees the child more occasionally who notices. That is why we ask you to write down other people's positive observations in the daily log. Even more proof that it is the wrong conclusion is that in our research, and so far we have followed children through two years of massage, the children of the parents who continued the daily massage for two years continued to make more even steady progress in development than those who didn't.

Hopefully this helps to head off a few problems at the pass!

Best wishes,

Louisa and Pam

Weekly Log - Week 44

♥ Always start with love

Check each day you do the massage

Sun ___ Mon ___ Tuesday ___ Wed ___ Thu ___ Fri ___ Sat ___

Things You Noticed:

During the Massage

Mv1. Lays down/won't lay down?

Mv2. Back – hums?

Mv3-4. Ears – avoids?

Mv5. Up/up/up – eye contact?

Mv6. Fingers – stroking or pressing?

Mv7. Chest – rubs eyes, yawns, relaxes?

Mv8. Belly – diarrhea/constipation?

Mv9-10. Legs – patting or pressing?

Mv11. Toes – stroking, pressing, bicycle?

Mv12. Soles – avoids?

During the Week

Sleep _____

Bowels _____

Tantrums _____

Affection _____

Eye contact _____

Listening _____

Speaking _____

Other_____

Positive things other people said about your child ...

Your thoughts and feelings about the process ...

Questions you had this week ...

Remember: Look for answers to your questions in the index and the book.

Week 45

Letter to parents – Sensory problems and success in school

Dear Parents,

We want to share what the massage has taught us about touch and other sensory problems in children with autism and what the implications are for school.

Why do schools pay so much attention to whether hearing and vision tests are normal? It's because they know that even mild hearing or vision impairment affects children's ability to learn. And severe impairment causes children to fall far behind in school. Educators want to make sure that sensory impairment is taken care of so children have the best chance of success in school.

While it is true that hearing and vision are very important, touch is even more important. Touch is the mother sense. It compensates for problems with the other senses, and it allows the brain to take in information from several senses at the same time. Deaf and blind children can develop their sense of touch to compensate for their loss. But when touch is abnormal, the nervous system becomes stressed, and hearing and vision can't compensate for touch. In fact, they become abnormal too. Noises seem too loud, lights seem too bright, and normal tastes and smells seem too strong. Without the organizing influence of touch, the senses stop working together. Sensory information becomes disorganized and confusing, and the child is easily overwhelmed. Not a good set-up for school.

But when touch problems are treated, the research shows that the nervous system calms down, and the other senses normalize right along with it.

So why aren't schools as concerned about abnormalities of touch? They should be. The touch and related sensory problems in autism are just as likely to result in lack of progress in school as hearing and vision impairment, probably more so.

Maybe part of the reason school officials aren't concerned is they don't realize that the touch and other sensory problems can be effectively treated. They know that hearing aids and glasses work for hearing and vision, they just don't know that there is a massage that works for sensory problems in autism. And neither do many parents.

But you do! So, please join us in getting the word out to families that you know that Qigong parent massage can help. Children with autism won't do well in school unless their sensory problems are treated. Research shows that their sensory problems are treatable. When touch problems are treated with qigong massage, the other sensory problems get better, behavior gets better, autism gets less severe, and children do better all around.

Nowadays, many children with autism are diagnosed by age three. The research shows that after one or two years of QST treatment, touch and other sensory problems can come down to normal. If parents start the massage with their three-year-olds, by the time they are old enough to go to school, they will have a much better chance of succeeding.

I guess you know we feel strongly about this! We really want all children to have the same chance that your child has now at succeeding in school.

All our best,

Louisa and Pam

PS. For those of you who are into science, go to, Appendix 1, Section 4. We will explain more about touch and the other senses. For the rest of you, just know that your massage is helping your child learn!

Weekly Log - Week 45

♥ Always start with love

Check each day you do the massage

Sun ___ Mon ___ Tuesday ___ Wed ___ Thu ___ Fri ___ Sat ___

Things You Noticed:

During the Massage

Mv1. Lays down/won't lay down?

Mv2. Back – hums?

Mv3-4. Ears – avoids?

Mv5. Up/up/up – eye contact?

Mv6. Fingers – stroking or pressing?

Mv7. Chest – rubs eyes, yawns, relaxes?

Mv8. Belly – diarrhea/constipation?

Mv9-10. Legs – patting or pressing?

Mv11. Toes – stroking, pressing, bicycle?

Mv12. Soles – avoids?

During the Week

Sleep _____

Bowels _____

Tantrums _____

Affection _____

Eye contact _____

Listening _____

Speaking _____

Other_____

Positive things other people said about your child ...

Your thoughts and feelings about the process ...

Questions you had this week ...

Remember: Look for answers to your questions in the index and the book.

Week 46

Letter to parents – Ann's story – autism and Down syndrome

Dear Parents,

I am blessed that I learned qigong massage. I always wish that I had learned it when my daughter Ann was two. My daughter was 18 years old when I took my first class in QST massage. That was ten years ago. Ann has both autism and Down syndrome. Her affection towards me amounted to presenting her forehead for me to kiss. She had difficulty feeding herself. At school she would hold the spoon, but was only able to bring it to her mouth if someone was physically touching her arm.

She had many sensory issues in her mouth and on her skin. Feeding her was difficult as she would be hungry, but the texture of the food was offensive to her. The first time I did the massage I did Movements 1 and 2 while she was standing. I was standing behind her. She brought her foot up and horse kicked me to the other side of the bathroom. Within two days she did not read the touch of the massage as a threat, and she would hand me her arm or leg, and lay still and enjoy the massage. Within one week of the massage she was feeding herself.

I also used it a lot for her diarrhea. She has had diarrhea on and off for years, and lots of problems with her colon. I always found that the massage would leave her stronger, and that when I was able to do it every day, the diarrhea backed off.

It has been ten years now since I started QST massage with her. She has now moved out of my home and into a home for disabled adults. I still use it on and off. Recently her eczema flared up, and I did it for a few weeks, and it all calmed down.

As an adult with Down syndrome and autism, I find that other people's expectations for my daughter are just that she maintain, not that she continue to learn and grow. But I feel like her brain has grown since I started the qigong massage. And I feel like it has improved the quality of her life. She has no speech, but she can communicate and make her wants and wishes known. And she can understand more of what others are saying.

The greatest gift of the massage was and is the bonding that takes place every time I do the massage and the affection she is able to show me now. She can give a full hug, and when excited to see me, will try to kiss me on my face.

If you have a child with Down syndrome and autism, and have a chance to start it early, I would totally recommend it. I think it could have made an even bigger difference if I could have started it at age two. As it is, I'm just grateful I have it now,

Sincerely,

Ann's Mom

Weekly Log - Week 46

♥ Always start with love

Check each day you do the massage

Sun ___ Mon ___ Tuesday ___ Wed ___ Thu ___ Fri ___ Sat ___

Things You Noticed:

During the Massage

Mv1. Lays down/won't lay down?

Mv2. Back – hums?

Mv3-4. Ears – avoids?

Mv5. Up/up/up – eye contact?

Mv6. Fingers – stroking or pressing?

Mv7. Chest – rubs eyes, yawns, relaxes?

Mv8. Belly – diarrhea/constipation?

Mv9-10. Legs – patting or pressing?

Mv11. Toes – stroking, pressing, bicycle?

Mv12. Soles – avoids?

During the Week

Sleep _____

Bowels _____

Tantrums _____

Affection _____

Eye contact _____

Listening _____

Speaking _____

Other_____

Positive things other people said about your child ...

Your thoughts and feelings about the process ...

Questions you had this week ...

Remember: Look for answers to your questions in the index and the book.

Week 47
Letter to parents – Helping other parents

Dear parents,

You've been using qigong massage with your child for about a year now, and you've likely seen quite a few improvements in your child, and your entire family is probably less stressed and confused and more relaxed as a result. One thing we've learned about parents of children with autism is that when they find something that works, they want to share it with other families and they want to learn more.

You have a lot to offer other families living with autism. You've been there. You learned qigong massage yourself, solved some challenges in the early weeks, learned how to adapt the massage to your child's changing needs, and hopefully you've gotten some encouragement and support in this first year from the letters in this workbook. You've probably seen improvements in lots of areas – sensory challenges, attention, sleep, digestion, meltdowns, transitions, language and social skills.

There are a number of ways you can share your experience with other families. You can connect with other families who have children with autism through your local schools, early childhood educators, special education teachers, and autism specialists. There may be local parent support organizations or groups for families with children with autism, and you can connect with other parents through them. State and national autism organizations such as the National Autism Association and Autism Speaks can also help you connect with other parents. And of course you can always give the gift of a book/DVD to a family you think could benefit from qigong massage.

If you're yearning to learn more about qigong massage yourself and go deeper, there are opportunities for you to do that, too. Did you know you can become a parent educator and teach qigong massage to other families and coach them as they get the massage into their family routine, just like you did? You can!

The Qigong Sensory Training Institute offers an online course for parents who want to learn to teach other parents to give the massage. In addition to the online learning, you'll support families by making weekly coaching visits for the first 12 weeks they're using the massage with their child at home. And you'll receive supervision and support from a Qigong Master Trainer the whole time. Then once you've successfully completed the course you can teach and support parents on your own. Of course you'll always have access to a Master Trainer when you need that support!

For more information on this course go to qsti.org and click on the Autism Professionals tab and the link to QST professional training (QST1 Parent Educator).

However you do it, you can share your experience with qigong massage and the hope you've found with other families, like someone may have shared it with you. Pass it on!

Best wishes,

Louisa and Pam

Weekly Log - Week 47

♥ Always start with love

Check each day you do the massage

Sun ___ Mon ___ Tuesday ___ Wed ___ Thu ___ Fri ___ Sat ___

Things You Noticed:

During the Massage

Mv1. Lays down/won't lay down?

Mv2. Back – hums?

Mv3-4. Ears – avoids?

Mv5. Up/up/up – eye contact?

Mv6. Fingers – stroking or pressing?

Mv7. Chest – rubs eyes, yawns, relaxes?

Mv8. Belly – diarrhea/constipation?

Mv9-10. Legs – patting or pressing?

Mv11. Toes – stroking, pressing, bicycle?

Mv12. Soles – avoids?

During the Week

Sleep _____

Bowels _____

Tantrums _____

Affection _____

Eye contact _____

Listening _____

Speaking _____

Other_____

Positive things other people said about your child ...

Your thoughts and feelings about the process ...

Questions you had this week ...

Remember: Look for answers to your questions in the index and the book.

Week 48
Letter to parents – Reflections from a brother and QST therapist

Dear parents,

I was two years old when my brother was born. There were some complications at birth, and he seemed to have problems right from the beginning. There was a new nervousness in our house that never really went away.

My brother was always the smallest kid in his age group. He had lots of ear infections. He looked dazed. I could feel how much he wanted to play with me, but his efforts were so disorganized. He drew strange pictures. He couldn't catch a ball. He didn't like hugs.

As he got older he was fascinated by the Marx brothers and liked to memorize presidential speeches. He could tell you the name of every restaurant in our town. Adults found him charming, but kids his age had no idea what to make of him.

As he discovered that other people thought he was strange and couldn't relate to his natural interests, my brother became increasingly withdrawn and aggressive. His teen years were really tough- on everyone. Toward the end of high school, my father told me, "I need you to look out for yourself a little here – we have our hands full with your brother.

He was finally able to move out of our parents' house into assisted living, and later on, out on his own. As an adult, he struggles, but he's had a series of jobs and has a girlfriend who seems very kind.

Over the past few years, I have shared Qigong massage with nearly 20 families with autism. I have witnessed more profound transformation that I thought possible in family after family. I have seen kids so disoriented they couldn't feel their feet become kids who could tie their own shoes. I have heard nine-year–olds speak their first words. I have seen kids who lived cowering in corners take roles in school plays. I have seen children who had been in such constant agony they could barely be touched sitting in a parent's lap playing patty-cake, maintaining eye contact, and laughing. And I have seen parents regain hope, recover their ability to connect with their kids, learn to read their kids' behavior, identify what their kids need, and learn how to provide it.

As I watch growth and hope and joy spread through the families I work with, I wonder what it would have been like for my brother and our family if we had known about QST. My brother needed someone to help him normalize touch so that hugs felt good, so that his body felt good, so that he could connect with other people in a healthy way. If he had gotten the massage when he was two or three years old, maybe he would have developed in a healthier, more normal way. I think he would have been more fluent in his social interactions. Other kids could have seen him as bright and creative instead of weird. He would have made friends.

It's painful to think about what would have been. But I know there is hope, because I have seen what is possible with Qigong massage. In sharing the massage with other families, I have healed every bit as much as any child or family I have worked with.

Jim

Weekly Log - Week 48

♥ Always start with love

Check each day you do the massage

Sun ___ Mon ___ Tuesday ___ Wed ___ Thu ___ Fri ___ Sat ___

Things You Noticed:

During the Massage

Mv1. Lays down/won't lay down?

Mv2. Back – hums?

Mv3-4. Ears – avoids?

Mv5. Up/up/up – eye contact?

Mv6. Fingers – stroking or pressing?

Mv7. Chest – rubs eyes, yawns, relaxes?

Mv8. Belly – diarrhea/constipation?

Mv9-10. Legs – patting or pressing?

Mv11. Toes – stroking, pressing, bicycle?

Mv12. Soles – avoids?

During the Week

Sleep _____

Bowels _____

Tantrums _____

Affection _____

Eye contact _____

Listening _____

Speaking _____

Other_____

Positive things other people said about your child ...

Your thoughts and feelings about the process ...

Questions you had this week ...

Remember: Look for answers to your questions in the index and the book.

Week 49
Letter to parents – Autism and seizures

Dear parents,

In our first book, we wrote that parents should not do the massage if their children had uncontrolled seizures. This is because, for some children with severe uncontrolled seizures, even light tapping on the head can actually provoke a seizure. If your child has severe uncontrolled seizures, we still recommend you do not start QST massage.

However, in the past five years of research, we have had the opportunity to do QST massage with a number of children with autism who had a mild seizure disorder for which they were on medication. They benefitted a lot from the massage, their autism became less severe, and they did not have seizures from the massage.

We did notice that their heads were more over-sensitive to touch than usual, and we developed a systematic approach to taking care of it.

If your child has mild seizure disorder which is controlled by medication, and you would like to start QST massage with them, here is what we recommend:

- For the first two weeks of the massage, start movements 1-4 in the standard location on the head. But instead of patting or pressing, gently stroke the head down to the neck in the direction of the movement. Pick up the patting or pressing at the neck and continue on down as your child prefers.

- If your child's head is too over-sensitive to tolerate stroking comfortably, then just start movements 1-4 at the neck and avoid the head altogether for a few weeks. Then try the stroking approach again to see if he tolerates it better.

- After several weeks of your child tolerating stroking on the head, substitute gentle pressure for the stroking movements on the head and continue from the neck down, as usual.

- After a month of using this gentle pressure, the sensitivity of the head should be improving. After three months using gentle pressure, it should be almost gone and you will likely be able to use patting or pressing from the beginning of each movement.

If at any time during this process your child becomes uncomfortable with stroking, pressing or patting, revert to the previous step for a few weeks until the head is no longer over-sensitive. For example, if your child is uncomfortable with stroking on the head, just start movements 1-4 at the neck and avoid the head for a few weeks before trying stroking again. If your child becomes uncomfortable with gentle pressing on the head, revert to stroking for a few weeks. And if your child becomes uncomfortable with patting/pressing, revert to gentle pressing for a few weeks until the head is no longer over-sensitive. Let your child's comfort level guide you in using this step-by-step process for treating over-sensitivity of the head.

Best wishes,

Louisa and Pam

Weekly Log - Week 49

♥ Always start with love

Check each day you do the massage

Sun ___ Mon ___ Tuesday ___ Wed ___ Thu ___ Fri ___ Sat ___

Things You Noticed:

During the Massage

Mv1. Lays down/won't lay down?

Mv2. Back – hums?

Mv3-4. Ears – avoids?

Mv5. Up/up/up – eye contact?

Mv6. Fingers – stroking or pressing?

Mv7. Chest – rubs eyes, yawns, relaxes?

Mv8. Belly – diarrhea/constipation?

Mv9-10. Legs – patting or pressing?

Mv11. Toes – stroking, pressing, bicycle?

Mv12. Soles – avoids?

During the Week

Sleep _____

Bowels _____

Tantrums _____

Affection _____

Eye contact _____

Listening _____

Speaking _____

Other_____

Positive things other people said about your child ...

Your thoughts and feelings about the process ...

Questions you had this week ...

Remember: Look for answers to your questions in the index and the book.

Week 50

Letter to parents – The importance of the self-regulation milestones in later life

Dear Parents,

Remember those self-regulation milestones that we learned about at the beginning of the year? Well, by now, your child is achieving them! He can face you and pay attention, he can sleep through the night, he can digest and eliminate regularly, and he can self-soothe. Congratulations! Every one of these milestones has come in because of your consistent work this year.

Now we'd like to show you what you have prevented from happening in your child's future. We said that the self-regulation milestones are the most important of the developmental milestones, and that if they were all delayed, the child would have autism. Now let's look at what happens when individual milestones are delayed, and how qigong massage can help.

Difficulty focusing and paying attention is very common in childhood, and is the main problem in attention deficit disorder (ADD). If the child is also hyper, it can result in attention deficit hyperactivity disorder (ADHD). That can mean decades of taking medication and managing side effects. Difficulty focusing and paying attention is also common in learning disorders of all kinds. We think much of this can be prevented or improved if parents start qigong massage as soon as the problem regulating attention is noticed. They would need to continue for a couple of years until the attention milestone is solidly in place.

Self-regulation of digestion and elimination. If the child does not achieve the ability to have regular digestion in the first few years of life, lifelong problems with diarrhea, constipation, reflux or irritable bowel syndrome can result. And they are at higher risk for food allergies, food intolerances and other chronic digestive conditions. Think about the number of adults who have these problems! What if they could be prevented in early childhood by daily qigong massage and careful attention to a clean and healthy diet? Wouldn't that be worth doing?

173

Self-regulation of sleep. There are countless stories of people who have never slept well – since early childhood. They have trouble falling asleep, don't stay asleep during the night, and don't wake up rested. Sound familiar? These were exactly the problems your child had when he started the massage. Qigong massage is a tremendous aid to the nervous system when it is establishing a good sleep-wake pattern. When parents also insist on a regular bed-time and don't allow video games in the evening, this is an excellent recipe for good sleep habits. And, by the way, those adults who don't rest well, also have problems with anxiety and chronic fatigue. Regular sleep is incredibly important to physical and mental health.

Self-soothing. Pediatricians' offices are full of children who do not self-soothe well. They are irritable, anxious, cry easily and have difficulties with tantrums. They are diagnosed with delays of behavioral self-regulation. Sometimes they are treated with attention to diet, and elimination of sugar, red dyes and processed foods. Sometimes, they are given medication from an early age. Once parents accept that their child needs medication to be calm, they are likely to keep it going for years. Although medication might artificially produce better behavior, it can't give the child their self-soothing milestone. As you have learned, that is only acquired through the sense of touch. And without their self-soothing milestone, children may turn to food to self-soothe. This can lead to problems with obesity. In their teenage years, children can also turn to alcohol, drugs or cigarettes to self-soothe. We believe that inability to self-soothe places children at risk for addictions of many kinds. How much better it would be to institute a program of daily qigong massage when the difficulty with self-soothing is first identified.

See what you've achieved, and what you've prevented? Congratulations!

All the best,

Louisa and Pam

Weekly Log - Week 50

♥ Always start with love

Check each day you do the massage

Sun ___ Mon ___ Tuesday ___ Wed ___ Thu ___ Fri ___ Sat ___

Things You Noticed:

During the Massage

Mv1. Lays down/won't lay down?

Mv2. Back – hums?

Mv3-4. Ears – avoids?

Mv5. Up/up/up – eye contact?

Mv6. Fingers – stroking or pressing?

Mv7. Chest – rubs eyes, yawns, relaxes?

Mv8. Belly – diarrhea/constipation?

Mv9-10. Legs – patting or pressing?

Mv11. Toes – stroking, pressing, bicycle?

Mv12. Soles – avoids?

During the Week

Sleep _____

Bowels _____

Tantrums _____

Affection _____

Eye contact _____

Listening _____

Speaking _____

Other_____

Positive things other people said about your child ...

Your thoughts and feelings about the process ...

Questions you had this week ...

Remember: Look for answers to your questions in the index and the book.

Week 51
Letter to parents – Year-end testing

Dear Parent,

Happy Anniversary! You've just completed your first year of Qigong parent massage. You did it, and you should feel very proud of yourself. It was tough at the beginning, but you persevered, and now you get to see just how much progress your child has made over the past year.

You'll recall that you completed two simple tests at the beginning of the year – the Autism Touch/Pain Checklist and the Autism Parenting Stress Index. Then you completed them again half way through the year to see how your child was progressing. You might remember that the Autism Touch/Pain Checklist measures how severe your child's touch/pain problems were and the Autism Parenting Stress index evaluates how challenging it is to parent your child. Now you will complete these tests a third time and see how the scores have continued to change the second half of the year.

Go ahead and complete the two simple tests, below, again. Then you can see just how much progress your child has made over the past year.

Autism Touch/Pain Checklist

Circle the response for each item that most accurately describes your child.

1. **Touch/Pain**	Often	Sometimes	Rarely	Never
• Does not cry tears when hurt	3	2	1	0
• Doesn't notice if the diaper is wet or dirty	3	2	1	0
• Face washing is difficult	3	2	1	0
• Haircuts are difficult	3	2	1	0
• Refuses to wear a hat	3	2	1	0
• Prefers to wear a hat	3	2	1	0
• Cutting fingernails is difficult	3	2	1	0
• Prefers to wear one or two gloves	3	2	1	0

• Avoids wearing gloves	3	2	1	0
• Cutting toenails is difficult	3	2	1	0
• Will only wear certain footwear (e.g. soft shoes, no socks)	3	2	1	0
• Prefers to wear the same clothes day after day	3	2	1	0
• Will only wear certain clothes (e.g. no elastic, no tags, only short pants)	3	2	1	0
• Cries tears when falls, scrapes skin or gets hurt (scale is reversed on purpose)	0	1	2	3
• Head bangs on a hard surface	3	2	1	0
• Head bangs on a soft surface	3	2	1	0

Add up the scores in each column: ___ ___ ___ ___

Add up the total score: _____

The Autism Parenting Stress Index

Please rate the following aspects of your child's health **according to how much stress it causes you and/or your family** by placing an X in the box that best describes your situation.	Not stressful	Sometimes creates stress	Often creates stress	Very stressful on a daily basis	So stressful at times I feel I cannot cope
Your child's ability to communicate					
Tantrums/meltdowns					
Aggressive behavior (siblings, peers)					
Self-injurious behavior					
Difficulty making transitions from one activity to another					
Sleep problems					
Your child's diet					
Bowel problems (diarrhea, constipation)					
Potty training					
Not feeling close to your child					
Concern for the future of your child being accepted by others					
Concern for the future of your child living independently					

Subtotal: _____   _____   _____   _____   _____

Total: _____

Now let's compare these scores with the scores from the same tests you completed back at the beginning and six months ago. Fill in the blanks, below:

First Autism Touch/Pain Checklist Total Score: _____

Mid-year Autism Touch/Pain Checklist Total Score: _____

Year-end Autism Touch/Pain Checklist Total Score: _____

First Autism Parenting Index Total Score: _____

Mid-year Autism Parenting Index Total Score: _____

Year-end Autism Parenting Index Total Score: _____

Did the scores continue to go down over the year? Depending on how severe your child's autism was to begin with, the scores may have come down a lot or a little. But they probably did come down. And this probably matches the improvements you are seeing in your child.

Your child's problems with touch have almost certainly improved. Even though there may still be some sensitivity in some areas, touch is becoming more normal. You're able to use parent touch a lot more now, and that is super important to your child's learning and development and his ability to connect with other people and the world around him.

And you are probably less stressed and more relaxed as a parent now than you were at the beginning, and maybe even more than you were 6 months ago.

So, it's time to celebrate! Sit back and enjoy hearing from a few parents who have traveled this journey before you.

> "Initially, I had low expectations of the massage. But as we continued, the changes were startling. Our little girl is more independent, dresses herself and goes to the bathroom alone! Boy, have our stress levels gone down: - Mother, 4 year old

> "Oh, it's made so much difference. My son is in school now, and I can't believe how well he's doing. Sure, he still has some challenges, but they're not nearly as big as before. - Dad, 7 year old

"Our son's teachers found his transformation remarkable, and wanted to learn more about the massage treatment." - Mother, 6 year old

"It's as if something has finally connected with her mind and body. Today I was moved to tears watching her play on the playground. She is so much more coordinated and she doesn't have to fight her body any more. She's in sync." - Mother, 5 year old

"Autism still confuses me, but I definitely believe in big possibilities now! She's improved so much already, I can't wait to see what the future holds for her." - Dad, 7 year old

Now write a sentence or two about your own experience with Qigong parent massage this past year:

Congratulations on your accomplishments.

Before you close out this workbook, we invite you to read our final thoughts to you below.

All our best,

Louisa and Pam

Weekly Log - Week 51

♥ Always start with love

Check each day you do the massage

Sun ___ Mon ___ Tuesday ___ Wed ___ Thu ___ Fri ___ Sat ___

Things You Noticed:

During the Massage

Mv1. Lays down/won't lay down?

Mv2. Back – hums?

Mv3-4. Ears – avoids?

Mv5. Up/up/up – eye contact?

Mv6. Fingers – stroking or pressing?

Mv7. Chest – rubs eyes, yawns, relaxes?

Mv8. Belly – diarrhea/constipation?

Mv9-10. Legs – patting or pressing?

Mv11. Toes – stroking, pressing, bicycle?

Mv12. Soles – avoids?

During the Week

Sleep _____

Bowels _____

Tantrums _____

Affection _____

Eye contact _____

Listening _____

Speaking _____

Other_____

Positive things other people said about your child ...

Your thoughts and feelings about the process ...

Questions you had this week ...

Remember: Look for answers to your questions in the index and the book.

Week 52
Letter to parents – Final thoughts and appreciations

Dear Parents,

We know that parenting children with autism requires a lot of extras – extra patience, extra courage, extra energy, extra stamina, extra hope, and extra support. We hope Qigong parent massage has provided you a little extra as the parent of a child with autism.

And now that you've come to the end of your first year with the massage, it's become a natural part of what you do as a family together. It's become a special time for you and your child. His behavior has improved, he is more connected to his body and the people and world around him. He is sleeping, eating and communicating better. And he is growing. You can hardly remember what a tantrum looks like – well, ok, even typically developing children occasionally melt down. But things are going much more smoothly and you are more relaxed as a parent. You are able to use much more touch with your child, and you know how important this is to learning and development.

So, let us ask you this: Why in the world would you want to stop doing the massage?! If you keep doing the massage, will it continue to help your child? Yes, it will! Will it support them as they navigate the normal rhythms, changes and challenges of life? Yes! Will it help them learn and develop? Yes! Will it support you in the challenging job of being a parent? Yes!

So, do you have to continue to give the massage every day forever? Well, no, not necessarily. But you might be interested to know that parents who keep it going five times a week have better outcomes than those who do it only a few days a week. Your child still needs extra help to get through the day. And when he doesn't get it, and he struggles to get through the day, those times tend to pile up in his system. Massage doesn't let things pile up. And keeping your child's system clear, clean and full with Qigong parent massage makes their engine run better, too, so they're more able to handle the demands of growing, developing and learning.

So, we hope you'll continue to use qigong massage with your child for as long as you feel it is supporting them and they're enjoying it.

> *"As for how it works, I don't know, I don't care, I just know that I've seen it work…and I'm sticking with it!" - Father*

You also have a lot to offer other parents who are just starting this journey. You can share your experience with others on Facebook.

We feel like we have traveled this road together with you as you started this adventure, struggled through the initial weeks, and gained skill and confidence. We have shared your joys as your child first looked you in the eye, said "I love you," let you hug him, or used the potty! We have shared your challenges and delight in your successes. We are so happy to have shared Qigong parent massage with you and your child. We wish you all the best as you continue to grow as a family.

We can't think of a better way to close than with the words of one 8-year-old child:

> *"Qigong is a special massage that I love and makes me feel good outside and inside and it helps me to be really balanced and smart. I love Qigong…you oughta try it."*

All our best as always,

Louisa and Pam

SECTION 4 - APPENDIXES

1. Information for Teachers

QST massage is a parent-delivered massage treatment for autism. Research studies confirm that when parents are trained and supported to give their children the daily massage, the severity of autism decreases by 32% in the first five months, and sensory problems decrease by 38%. The massage is a sensory treatment for autism. It is a form of massage known as qigong massage, that is based on Eastern medicine and is focused on normalizing children's response to touch and improving child-to-parent bonding and interactions.

Sensory difficulties in autism cause behavioral difficulties and learning delays in the classroom. QST massage is an effective sensory treatment for autism that results in improved classroom behavior, and improved child ability to focus, listen and learn in the classroom environment. Studies have shown that sensory impairment must be remediated in order for children to fully benefit from their educational program.

This program is recommended for early intervention for autism at the time of autism diagnosis. It has been shown to decrease the severity of autism, increase receptive communication and improve behavioral self-regulation. It improves children's ability to benefit from early intervention classroom programs.

For more information for parents, and for the parent-training guide Qigong Massage for Your Child with Autism: A Home Program from Chinese Medicine, see www.qsti.org.

References:

Articles can be downloaded from www.qsti.org.

1. Early intervention with a parent-delivered massage protocol directed at tactile abnormalities decreases severity of autism and improves child-to-parent interactions: a replication study. Autism Research and Treatment.

2. Treatment of Tactile Impairment in Young Children with Autism: Results with Qigong Massage. Silva, L. Schalock, M. (2013). International Journal of Therapeutic

Massage and Bodywork, 6(4):12-20.

3. Prevalence and Significance of Abnormal Tactile Responses in Young Children with Autism. Silva, L. Schalock, M. (2013). North American Journal of Medicine and Science, 6(3):121-127.

4. Early Intervention for Autism with a Parent-delivered Qigong Massage Program: A Randomized Controlled Trial. Silva, L., Schalock, M. & Gabrielsen, K. (2011). American Journal of Occupational Therapy, 65(5):550-559.

5. Qigong Massage Treatment for Sensory and Self-Regulation Problems in Young Children with Autism: A Randomized Controlled Trial . Silva, L., Schalock, M., Ayres, R., Bunse, C., & Budden, S. (2009). American Journal of Occupational Therapy, 63, 423-432.

2. Information for your child's doctor

QST massage is a parent-delivered massage treatment for autism. Research studies confirm that when parents are trained and supported to give their children the daily massage, the severity of autism decreases by 32% in the first five months, sensory problems decrease by 38%, and parenting stress decreases by 44%. The massage is a sensory treatment for autism. It is a form of massage known as qigong massage that is based on Eastern medicine that is focused on normalizing children's response to touch and improving child-to-parent bonding and interactions.

Almost 100% of children with autism respond abnormally to touch. Parent touch is critical to early development. Parenting stress for parents of young children with autism is four times greater than typically developing children. No other program has reported the large decreases in parenting stress reported by this program. With normalization of touch, child-to-parent interactions improve, children become more receptive and affectionate, and development improves.

This program is recommended for early intervention for autism at the time of autism diagnosis.

For more information for parents, and for the parent-training guide Qigong Massage for Your Child with Autism: A Home Program from Chinese Medicine, see www.qsti.org.

References:

Articles can be downloaded from www.qsti.org.

1. Early intervention with a parent-delivered massage protocol directed at tactile abnormalities decreases severity of autism and improves child-to-parent interactions: a replication study. Autism Research and Treatment.

2. Treatment of Tactile Impairment in Young Children with Autism: Results with Qigong Massage. Silva, L. Schalock, M. (2013). International Journal of Therapeutic Massage and Bodywork, 6(4):12-20.

3. Prevalence and Significance of Abnormal Tactile Responses in Young Children with Autism. Silva, L. Schalock, M. (2013). North American Journal of Medicine and Science, 6(3):121-127.

4. Early Intervention for Autism with a Parent-delivered Qigong Massage Program: A Randomized Controlled Trial. Silva, L., Schalock, M. & Gabrielsen, K. (2011). American Journal of Occupational Therapy, 65(5):550-559.

5. Qigong Massage Treatment for Sensory and Self-Regulation Problems in Young Children with Autism: A Randomized Controlled Trial . Silva, L., Schalock, M., Ayres, R., Bunse, C., & Budden, S. (2009). American Journal of Occupational Therapy, 63, 423-432.

INDEX

Made in the USA
Coppell, TX
18 April 2024

31450206R00107